Official

General Medicine Word Games

Jannet Books & Publishing presents General Medicine Word Games. Awaiting you in these pages are more than 50 fun-filled games. These fun-filled games include forming plural nouns, finding adjectives, finding abbreviations and more.

We would love to get your feedback about General Medicine Word Games. Follow the author on social media.

Facebook: Dharamdat Sumare

Instagram: _doctor_entrepreneur_

YouTube: Doctor Entrepreneur

Twitter: @doctorentrepre1

ISBN: 978-976-96145-2-9

Disclaimer

The purpose of this book is for entertainment only. It should NOT be used for diagnosing or treating patients. The author and associates take no responsibility for misusing this book for any purposes other than entertainment. The games in this book are the property of the author. No part of this book should be used without the authorization of the author(s) or JANNET BOOKS & JANNET PUBLISHING.

Published & Distributed by:
Jannet Books & Publishing
41 University Crescent
Kingston 10
St. Andrew
Jamaica
Email: jannetbooks@yahoo.com

Published July 6, 2018

ISBN: 978 976 96145 2 9

I Dedicate This Book My Mother

She was a leader who was second to none.

She was a lioness who hunted for her pride.

She was a warrior who had no limits.

She was a heroine who won every battle because she never gave up.

She was a queen who wore the oldest of clothing, so that her children could dress like princes and princesses.

She was a desi who wore no shoes so that her children could wear.

She was a mother who walked a thousand miles so that her children would walk one.

She was a commander-in-chief who took her family out of poverty and placed them on the path of success.

She was a woman who loved God above all.

Rest in peace mom.

Your loving son.

Dr. Dharamdat Sumare

Instruction

Please read all the instructions.

Locate the puzzle words on the grid. The words can run in any one of the eight directions. Some of the unused letters are clues to solve the Mega Puzzle, Bonus Puzzle and other Puzzles.

Plural nouns
BURSAE
SCAPULAE
VERTEBRAE
VENAE CAVAE
LARVAE
CONJUNCTIVAE
PETECHIAE
AXILLAE
SCLERAE

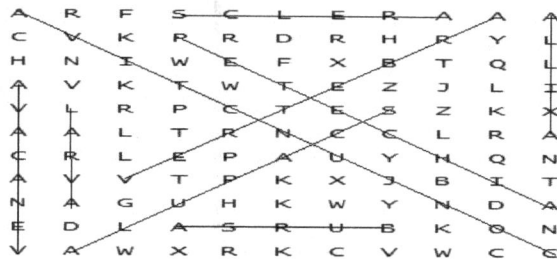

Need help? Solve Puzzle # ...
Give up? Solution is on Page. ...

Puzzle words

Note the changes made before the words are located on the grid.

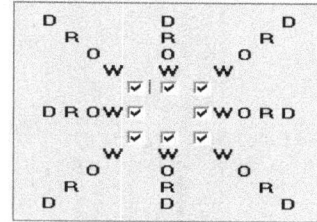

Grid

Mega Puzzle clue
1st Four unused letters
__ * __ * __ * __
  1   2   3   4

Direction of words
Letters to be placed in Mega Puzzle

Clues & Answers

Word Search: Chapters 1, 2, 3, 5,16 & Part of 12.

Solve the puzzle the same way that you'd solve a numeric sudoku. Each of the letters A, B C, D, E, F, G, H, I, J, K, L, M, N, O, P, Q, R, S, T, U, V, Q, X and Y is found once in every row, column and 5×5 box.

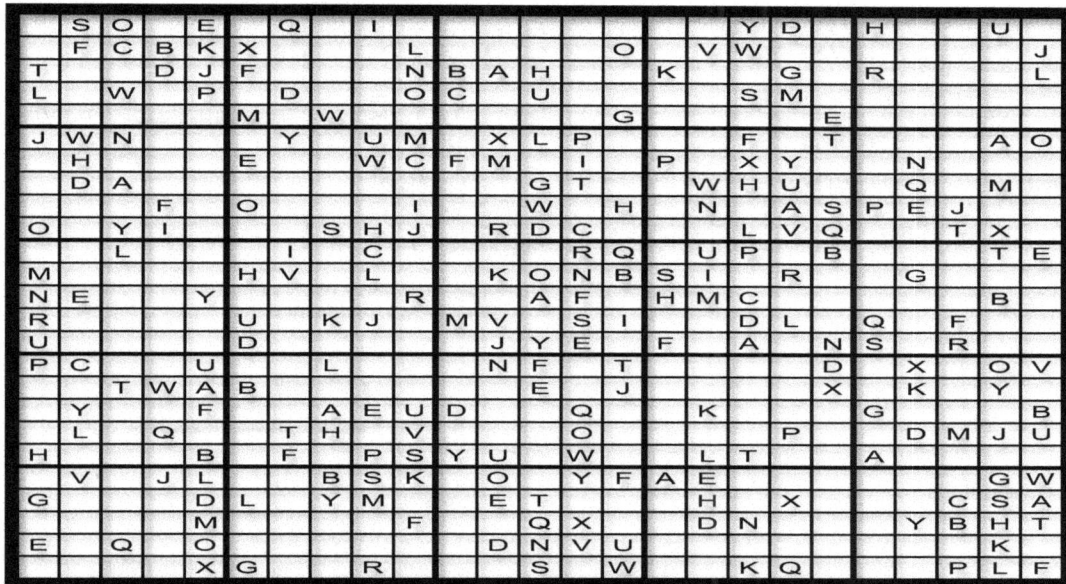

Chapter 4: Letter Sudoku

INSTRUCTIONS

Follow the arrows to find the answers. Each answer has four clues; the no of letters, the first and last letter, and a specification.

1st clue : # of letters, 1st letter & Last letter
2 nd Clue
Specific to the word

Play area

Mega Puzzle clue
1st Four unused letters
__ * __ * __ * __
1   2   3   4

Need help? Solve Puzzle # ...
Give up? Solution is on Page ...

Letters to be placed in Mega Puzzle

Clues & Answers

Chapters 13 & 14: Clues in Squares

For puzzle # 28, scan the grid in all directions for the 15 nine-letter words in the shape of a G. For puzzle # 29, scan the grid in all directions for the eleven pairs of 5 letter words in form of a X or +.

X & + search
CHEST X CLEFT .

G search
PATHOLOGY

Puzzle words

Play area

Mega Puzzle clue
1st Four unused letters
__ * __ * __ * __
1   2   3   4

Need help? Solve Puzzle # ...
Give up? Solution is on Page ...

Letters to be placed in Mega-puzzle

Clues & Answers

Chapter 7: Nine & Five Letters Word Search

Enter the letters in the grid according to the corresponding numbers until the missing letters and the words are revealed.

Grid clues

15	21	17	20	12	16
A	S	T	H	M	A

Play area

1	2	3	4	5	6	7	8	9	10	11	12	13
E			C			N					M	
14	15	16	17	18	19	20	21	22	23	24	25	26
A	P	T	O	H	S	U	I	B	G	L		

Need help? Solve Puzzle # ...
Give up? Solution is on Page ...

Mega Puzzle clue
1st Four unused letters
_ * _ * _ * _ *
1   2   3   4

Letters to be placed in Mega Puzzle

Clues & Answers

Chapter 15: Coded

To solve this puzzle, use unbroken lines in which the last letter of one abbreviation is the first or last letter of the next abbreviation. Find your way through the puzzle to the finish line.

Puzzle abbreviations

1. N S T E M I
2. _ _ _ _
3. _ _ _ _ _
4. _ _ _ _
5. _ _ _ _
6. _ _ _ _
7. _ _ _ _
8. _ _ _ _
9. _ _ _ _
10. _ _ _ _

Start/ Finish

Play area

Need help? Solve Puzzle # ...
Give up? Solution is on Page ...

Mega Puzzle clue
1st Four unused letters
_ * _ * _ * _ *
1   2   3   4

Letters to be placed in Mega Puzzle

Clues & Answers

Chapter 6: Tail Tag

INSTRUCTIONS

Some of the puzzles contain clues that are used to complete the Mega Puzzle. These clues are only available on completion of the puzzles from page 5 to 54. Some of these clues include, but not limited to: first used letter, first unused letter, last unused letter, the most crossed/intersected letter...etc.

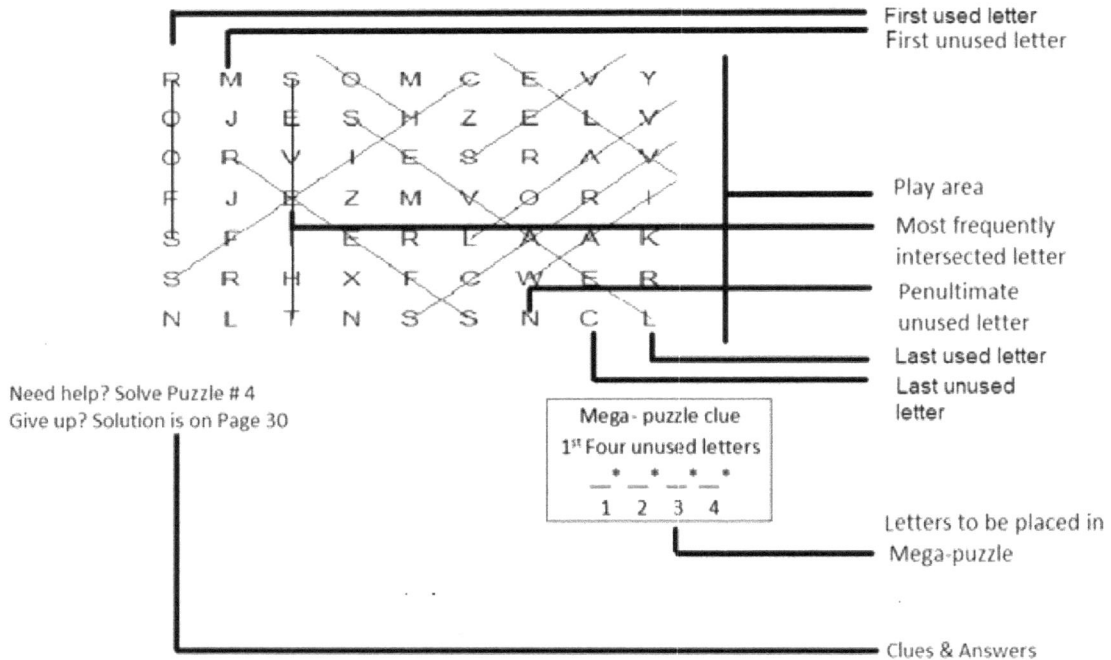

First used letter
First unused letter

R M S O M C E V Y
O J E S H Z E L V
O R V I E S R A V
F J E Z M V O R I
S F E R L A K
S R H X F C W E R
N L T N S S N C L

Play area

Most frequently intersected letter

Penultimate unused letter

Last used letter

Last unused letter

Need help? Solve Puzzle # 4
Give up? Solution is on Page 30

Mega- puzzle clue
1st Four unused letters
_ * _ * _ * _ *
1   2   3   4

Letters to be placed in Mega-puzzle

Clues & Answers

Chapter 1: Mega Puzzle

Contents

Author:

Dr. Dharamdat Sumare

Cover Designer:

Dr. Dharamdat Sumare

Graphic Designer

Dr. Dharamdat Sumare

Mega Puzzle

The objective of General Medicine Word Games is to complete the Mega-Puzzle. The Mega Puzzle contains 3 puzzles:

Firstly, one of the longest documented word (in dictionaries) which is a forty-five letter terminology is the starting of the Mega Puzzle. To finish this puzzle, complete the puzzles on pages 5 to 67 to uncover clues that will assist.

Secondly, there are 26 carefully selected words that are formed using the letters from the forty-five letter terminology (the first part of the Mega puzzle). To finish this puzzle, complete the puzzles on pages 5 to 67 to uncover clues that will assist.

Lastly, complete the word search game on page # 3.

Note: The missing letters for the words of the Mega Puzzle are numbered from 1 to 331. Complete the puzzles on pages 5 to 57 to uncover clues to assist in the completion of the Mega Puzzle.

Please see the instructions for more information or visit our YouTube and watch the videos.

Important: The solution to the Mega Puzzle is not found in this book. However, it can be obtained on social media.
Facebook: Dharamdat Sumare

Instagram: _doctor_entrepreneur_

YouTube: Doctor Entrepreneur

Twitter: @doctorentrepre1

         U

___ ___
1   2   3   4   5   6   7   8   9 10 11 12 13 14 15 16 17 18 19 20 21 22 23 24 25

___ ___ ___ ___ ___ ___ ___ ___ ___ ___ ___ ___ ___ ___ ___ ___ ___ ___ ___ ___
26 27 28 29 30 31 32 33 34 35 36 37 38 39 40 41 42 43 44 45

Seventeen letter words

___ ___ ___ ___ ___ ___ ___ ___ ___ ___ ___ ___ ___ ___ ___ ___ ___
46 47 48 49 50 51 52 53 54 55 56 57 58 59 60 61 62
                             I
___ ___ ___ ___ ___ ___ ___ ___ ___ ___ ___ ___ ___ ___ ___ ___ ___
63 64 65 66 67 68 69 70 71 72 73 74 75 76 77 78 79

Sixteen letter words

___ ___ ___ ___ ___ ___ ___ ___ ___ ___ ___ ___ ___ ___ ___ ___
80 81 82 83 84 85 86 87 88 89 90 91 92 93 94 95

___ ___ ___ ___ ___ ___ ___ ___ ___ ___ ___ ___ ___ ___ ___ ___
96 97 98 99 100 101 102 103 104 105 106 107 108 109 110 111

Fifteen letter words

___ ___ ___ ___ ___ ___ ___ ___ ___ ___ ___ ___ ___ ___ ___
112 113 114 115 116 117 118 119 120 121 122 123 124 125 126

___ ___ ___ ___ ___ ___ ___ ___ ___ ___ ___ ___ ___ ___ ___
127 128 129 130 131 132 133 134 135 136 137 138 139 140 141

Fourteen letter words

                                              A
___ ___ ___ ___ ___ ___ ___ ___ ___ ___ ___ ___ ___ ___ ___
142 143 144 145 146 147 148 149 150 151 152 153 154 155

___ ___ ___ ___ ___ ___ ___ ___ ___ ___ ___ ___ ___ ___
156 157 158 159 160 161 162 163 164 165 166 167 168 169

Thirteen letter words

___ ___ ___ ___ ___ ___ ___ ___ ___ ___ ___ ___ ___
170 171 172 173 174 175 176 177 178 179 180 181 182

___ ___ ___ ___ ___ ___ ___ ___ ___ ___ ___ ___ ___
183 184 185 186 187 188 189 190 191 192 193 194 195

Twelve letter words

___ ___ ___ ___ ___ ___ ___ ___ ___ ___ ___ ___
196 197 198 199 200 201 202 203 204 205 206 207

___ ___ ___ ___ ___ ___ ___ ___ ___ ___ ___ ___
208 209 210 211 212 213 214 215 216 217 218 219

Eleven letter words

___ ___ ___ ___ ___ ___ ___ ___ ___ ___ ___
220 221 222 223 224 225 226 227 228 229 230

                                    S
___ ___ ___ ___ ___ ___ ___ ___ ___ ___ ___
231 232 233 234 235 236 237 238 239 240 241

Ten letter words

___ ___ ___ ___ ___ ___ ___ ___ ___ ___
242 243 244 245 246 247 248 249 250 251
                                   R
___ ___ ___ ___ ___ ___ ___ ___ ___ ___
252 253 254 255 256 257 258 259 260 261

Nine letter words

                          R
___ ___ ___ ___ ___ ___ ___ ___ ___
262 263 264 265 266 267 268 269 270

___ ___ ___ ___ ___ ___ ___ ___ ___
271 272 273 274 275 276 277 278 279

Eight letter words

___ ___ ___ ___ ___ ___ ___ ___
280 281 282 283 284 285 286 287

___ ___ ___ ___ ___ ___ ___ ___
288 289 290 291 292 293 294 295

Seven letter words

___ ___ ___ ___ ___ ___ ___
296 297 298 299 300 301 302

___ ___ ___ ___ ___ ___ ___
303 304 305 306 307 308 309

Six letter words

___ ___ ___ ___ ___ ___
310 311 312 313 314 315

___ ___ ___ ___ ___ ___
316 317 318 319 320 321

Five letter words

___ ___ ___ ___ ___
322 323 324 325 326

___ ___ ___ ___ ___
327 328 329 330 331

Mega Puzzle

LOCATE THE ABOVE WORDS ON THE GRID TO CHECK FOR ACCURACY.

```
C C O O A C I T A I C S N N G R N A U
L A U T S P M U M S U S L O A O S C L
A R T N I T O M E N U N S I I J I I T
S C R P C W E R U R B T N S X L S P R
U I F W T O O O I L E Q S S F L O O A
A N N Y L S N V M O U I G E F E R C M
P O J O A E O S S A M C C R T P E S I
O M L N I I S A C S P A E P J T L O C
N A M E L T R A N I N N C P N O C R R
E T L O C C C A P A O I N U S S S A O
M O P F O R R U L I R U X S N P O P S
T S B M J T A I S E L Q S O N I T A C
S I A N O P C N T O R X L N T R O L O
O S F R B U T C O Q P O Q U E O R R P
P W U G L H I F X N C I B M X S Z N E
T E Q I C O R P O R E A L M T I S N Q
N Q R O S S E R P O S A V I P S B T K
K G M I C R O V A S C U L A T U R E N
F T V M I C R O C I R C U L A T I O N
```

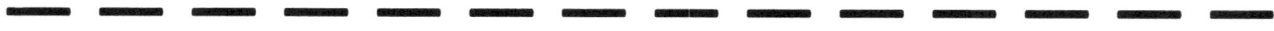

- - - - - - - - - - - - - - - - -

The 1st fourteen unused letters reveal a message

Chapter 2

Singular & Plural

Medical nouns do not follow the rules in English Language to form their plural. Therefore, I have researched and created some rules to aid doctors and students to make the task of forming plural medical nouns less difficult.

Important to remember: Some medical nouns have more than one plural forms. I have used the simplest form to avoid confusion.

Example:

condyloma (singular form): condylomata & condylomas (plural forms)

Rule # 1. Some singular medical nouns that end with *a* are pluralized by dropping the *a* and adding *ae*.

Example: *a*   axill*a*   *ae*   axill*ae*

LOCATE ON THE GRID, THE PLURAL FOR EACH LISTED SINGULAR NOUN.

Singular nouns

~~AXILLA~~

CONJUNCTIVA

VERTEBRA

SCLERA

PETECHIA

LARVA

SCAPULA

BURSA

VENA CAVA

N	X	V	E	R	T	E	B	R	A	E	D
E	A	V	I	T	C	N	U	J	N	O	C
E	V	C	T	E	J	Y	W	E	L	Q	M
A	L	E	B	G	A	G	A	K	G	P	M
S	T	A	N	W	F	L	X	K	E	P	J
R	P	R	K	A	U	Q	L	T	H	T	F
U	C	E	L	P	E	T	E	I	W	L	G
B	R	L	A	G	J	C	H	N	X	Z	B
D	R	C	R	M	H	P	A	N	R	A	N
R	S	S	V	I	K	T	M	V	N	M	G
L	H	L	A	M	T	C	D	N	A	R	H
K	T	E	E	R	M	N	P	K	Y	E	R

LOCATE ON THE GRID, THE SINGULAR FOR EACH LISTED PLURAL NOUN.

Plural nouns

BURSAE

SCAPULAE

VERTEBRAE

VENAE CAVAE

LARVAE

CONJUNCTIVAE

PETECHIAE

AXILLAE

SCLERAE

A	R	F	S	C	L	E	R	A	A	A
C	V	K	P	R	D	R	H	R	Y	L
H	N	I	W	E	F	X	B	T	Q	L
A	V	K	T	W	T	E	Z	J	L	I
V	L	R	P	C	T	E	S	Z	K	X
A	A	L	T	R	N	C	C	L	R	A
C	R	L	E	P	A	U	Y	H	Q	N
A	V	V	T	P	K	X	J	B	I	T
N	A	G	U	H	K	W	Y	N	D	A
E	D	L	A	S	R	U	B	K	O	N
V	A	W	X	R	K	C	V	W	C	C

MEGA PUZZLE CLUE
The last unused letter on grid 1a is the letter for the Mega Puzzle
12, 17, 56, 66, 69, 83, 94 & 99.

Give up? Solutions are on Pages 69 & 77.

Rule # 2. Some singular medical nouns that end with *is* are pluralized by dropping the *is* and
adding *es.*

Example:

is   arthro*is*   *es*   arthros*es*

Exception to the rule:

is   epididym*is*   *ides*   epididym*ides*

LOCATE ON THE GRID, THE PLURAL FOR EACH LISTED SINGULAR NOUN.

Singular nouns

ARTHROSIS
NEUROSIS
ANALYSIS
DIAGNOSIS
EXOSTOSIS
PROGNOSIS
METASTASIS
TESTIS
PELVIS
EXCEPTIONS:
EPIDIDYMIS
IRIS
HEPATITIS

K	E	P	I	D	I	D	Y	M	I	D	E	S	H
K	R	X	R	E	X	O	S	T	O	S	E	S	D
G	Y	P	B	S	L	H	P	J	E	K	X	E	I
F	H	R	R	T	E	D	J	D	B	N	N	S	A
X	E	L	P	O	K	V	I	Q	E	L	Q	O	G
F	P	T	G	Z	G	R	L	U	V	S	J	R	N
L	A	N	K	R	I	N	R	E	E	N	H	O
Y	T	S	L	R	Z	O	O	S	P	T	R	T	S
R	I	E	B	Q	S	D	Y	S	K	T	P	R	E
X	T	T	R	E	R	L	W	V	E	K	T	A	S
G	I	S	S	T	A	G	N	P	K	S	Z	P	C
X	D	E	R	N	R	K	C	X	L	V	C	N	M
C	E	T	A	H	H	Z	M	R	G	R	Q	W	G
Y	S	S	E	S	A	T	S	A	T	E	M	N	H

LOCATE ON THE GRID, THE SINGULAR FOR EACH LISTED PLURAL NOUN.

Plural nouns

ARTHROSES
ANALYSES
EXOSTOSES
PROGNOSES
DIAGNOSES
NEUROSES
METASTASES
PELVES
TESTES
EXCEPTIONS:
IRIDES
EPIDIDYMIDES
HEPATITIDES

N	S	I	S	A	T	S	A	T	E	M	K
Z	M	N	M	A	N	A	L	Y	S	I	S
W	D	D	S	F	Y	L	J	I	F	W	S
E	P	I	K	I	W	P	S	X	H	X	I
X	R	B	A	L	T	O	T	E	M	S	S
O	O	J	M	G	R	S	P	K	S	I	O
S	G	Y	K	U	N	A	E	I	T	V	R
T	N	H	E	C	T	O	R	T	J	L	H
O	O	N	L	I	G	I	S	W	P	E	T
S	S	V	T	W	N	T	Q	I	J	P	R
I	I	I	T	B	Y	T	T	M	S	Y	A
S	S	S	I	M	Y	D	I	D	I	P	E

MEGA PUZZLE CLUE
The last letter on grid 2b is the Mega Puzzle letter for # 226,
264, 277, 290, 299, 306, 311 & 321.

Give up? Solutions are on Pages 69 & 77

Rule # 3. Some singular nouns that end with *ex or ix* are pluralized by replacing the endings with
ices.

Examples:	*ex*	cort*ex*	*ices*	cort*ices*
	ix	cerv*ix*	*ices*	cerv*ices*

Singular nouns: INDEX   CORTEX   VARIX   CERVIX   APPENDIX   FORNIX

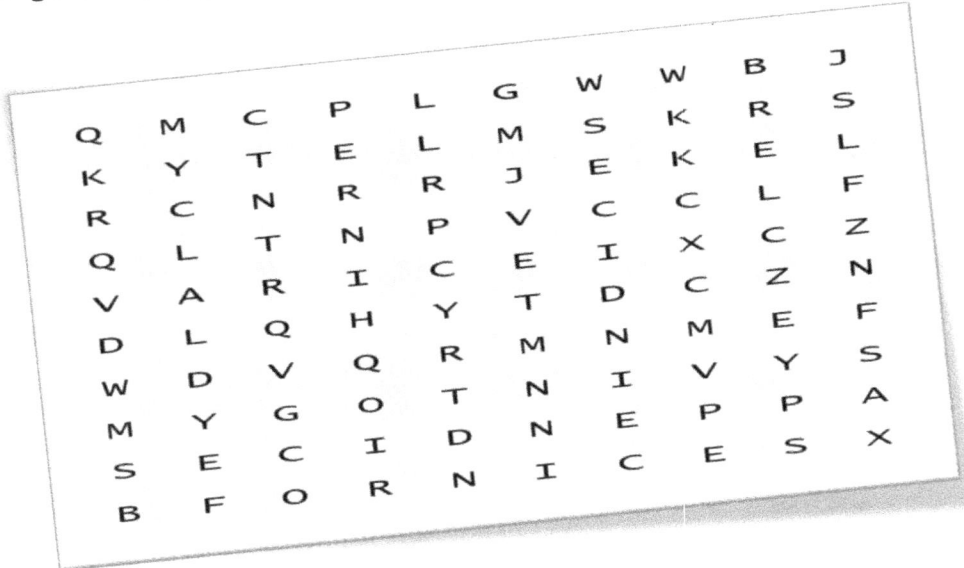

LOCATE ON THE GRID, THE PLURAL FOR EACH LISTED SINGULAR NOUN.

Q   M   C   P   L   G   W   W   B   J
K   Y   T   E   L   M   S   K   R   S
R   C   N   R   R   J   E   K   E   L
Q   L   T   N   P   V   C   C   L   F
V   A   R   I   C   E   I   X   C   Z
D   L   Q   H   Y   T   D   C   Z   N
W   D   V   Q   R   M   N   M   E   F
M   Y   G   O   T   N   I   V   Y   S
S   E   C   I   D   N   E   P   P   A
B   F   O   R   N   I   C   E   S   X

Plural nouns: INDICES   CORTICES   VARICES   CERVICES   APPENDICES   FORNICES.

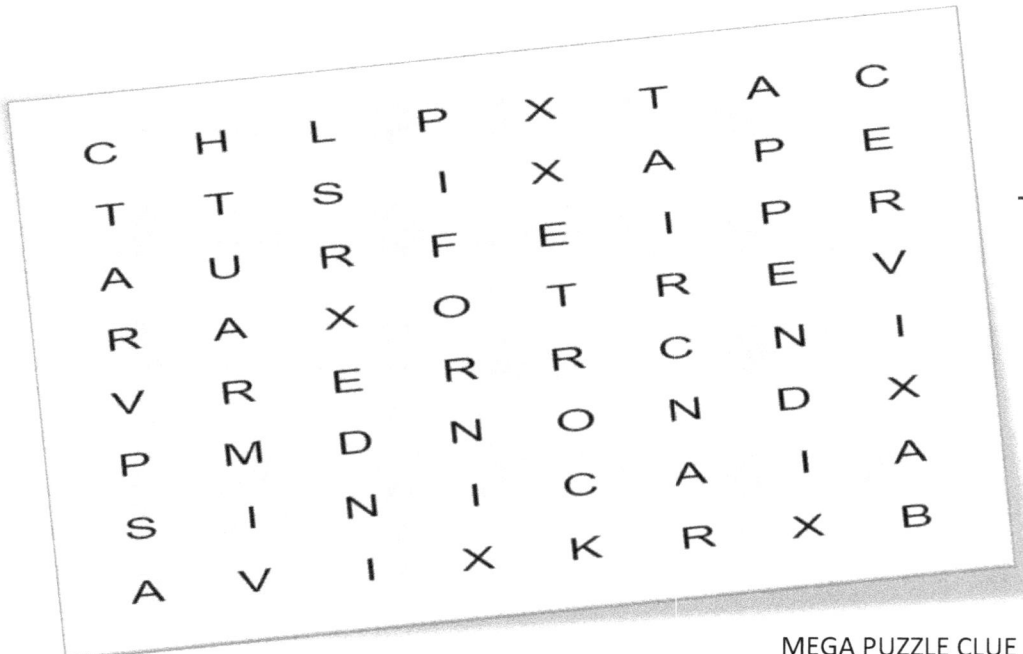

LOCATE ON THE GRID, THE SINGULAR FOR EACH LISTED PLURAL NOUN.

C   H   L   P   X   T   A   C
T   T   S   I   X   A   P   E
A   U   R   F   E   I   P   R
R   A   X   O   T   R   E   V
V   R   E   R   R   C   N   I
P   M   D   N   O   N   D   X
S   I   N   I   C   A   I   A
A   V   I   X   K   R   X   B

MEGA PUZZLE CLUE
The most intersected letter on grid 3a is the letter for the Mega
Puzzle # 97, 102, 109, 119, 133, 160, 168, 190, 194 & 206.

Give up?   olutions are on Pages 69 & 77

7

Rule # 4. Some singular medical nouns that end with *ma* are pluralized by adding *ta*.
Example: *ma*   adeno*ma*   *ta*   adenoma*ta*

Singular nouns   *LOCATE ON THE GRID, THE PLURAL FOR EACH LISTED SINGULAR NOUN.*

ADENOMA

CARCINOMA

CONDYLOMA

FIBROMA

LEIOMYOMA

SARCOMA

STOMA

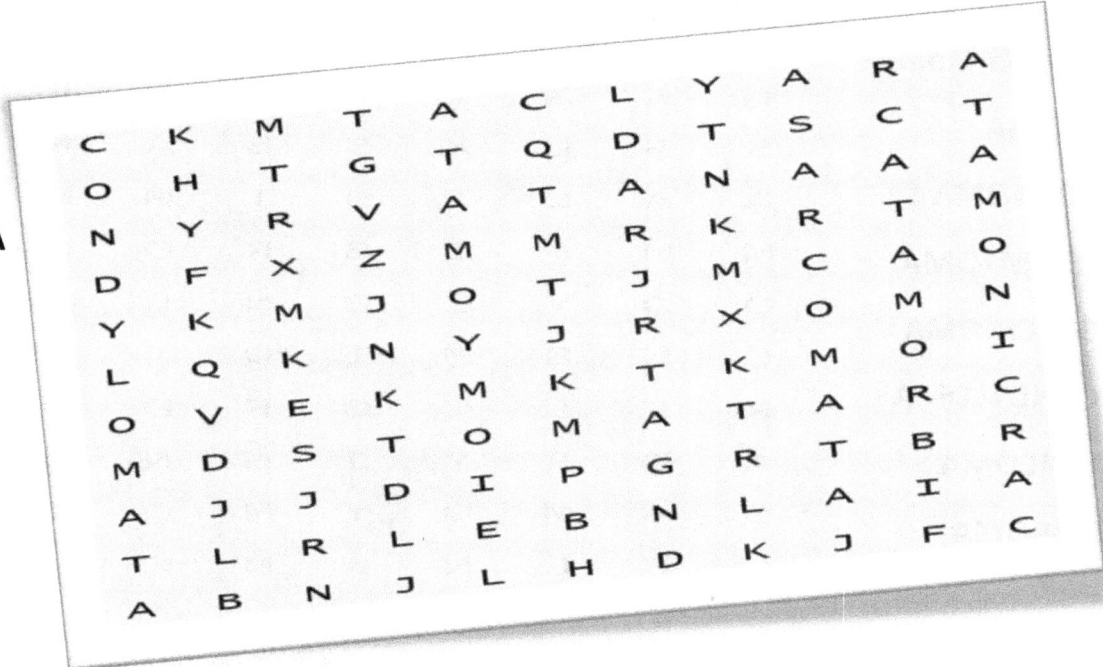

Plural nouns   *LOCATE ON THE GRID, THE SINGULAR FOR EACH LISTED PLURAL NOUN.*

LEIOMYOMATA

CARCINOMATA

ADENOMATA

CONDYLOMATA

STOMATA

FIBROMATA

SARCOMATA

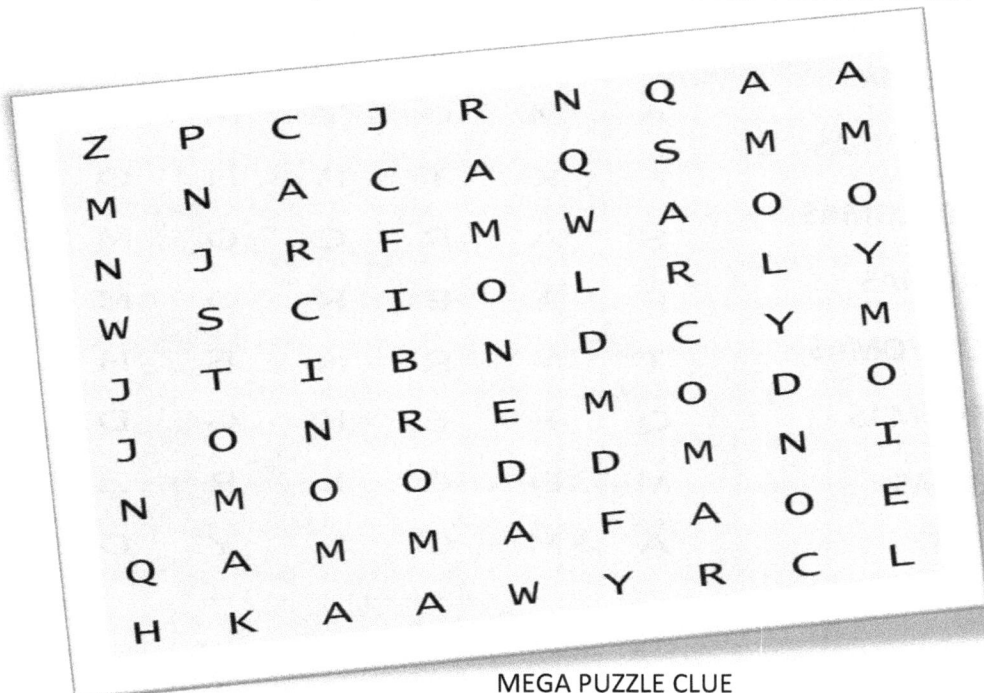

MEGA PUZZLE CLUE
The last unused letter on grid 4b is the letter for Mega Puzzle # 103, 130, 135, 158, 177, 191, 200, 215, 225 & 230.

Give up? Solutions are on Pages 69 & 77

8

Some singular medical nouns that end with *ma* are pluralized by adding *s* as the English rule.
Example:

ma   adeno*ma*   *s*   adenoma*s*

LOCATE ON THE GRID, THE PLURAL FOR EACH LISTED SINGULAR NOUN.

Singular nouns

STOMA

ADENOMA

LEIOMYOMA

CARCINOMA

CONDYLOMA

SARCOMA

FIBROMA

L	K	X	Y	X	R	S	B	Y	S
S	S	L	X	S	B	A	N	A	G
A	A	L	T	H	T	M	M	R	J
M	M	F	I	B	R	O	M	A	S
O	O	Y	C	B	N	L	M	D	N
C	N	B	M	I	Q	Y	N	A	N
R	E	L	C	Q	F	D	D	F	S
A	D	R	Y	J	G	N	N	L	L
S	A	M	O	Y	M	O	I	E	L
C	B	L	N	W	M	C	V	P	Y

LOCATE ON THE GRID, THE SINGULAR FOR EACH PLURAL NOUN.

Plural nouns

ADENOMAS

CARCINOMAS

CONDYLOMAS

FIBROMAS

LEIOMYOMAS

SARCOMAS

STOMAS

C	A	R	C	I	N	O	M	A
A	M	O	Y	M	O	I	E	L
F	K	T	B	H	Q	A	N	B
S	A	R	C	O	M	A	B	A
F	I	B	R	O	M	A	N	M
T	M	R	N	F	H	P	T	O
Q	F	E	K	G	D	C	X	T
M	D	C	L	R	Z	R	N	S
A	M	O	L	Y	D	N	O	C

MEGA PUZZLE CLUE
The most intersected letter on grid 5a is the Mega Puzzle letter for #
Give up? Solutions are on Pages 69 ,70 & 77   30, 32, 37, 39, 42, 51, 61, 67, 78, 84 & 100.

Rule # 5. Some singular medical nouns that end with *nx* are pluralized by dropping the endings *x*
and adding *ges*.

Example: *nx*   lary*nx*   *ges*   laryn*ges*

Singular nouns   **LOCATE ON THE GRID, THE PLURAL FOR EACH SINGULAR NOUN.**

LARYNX

PHALANX

MENINX

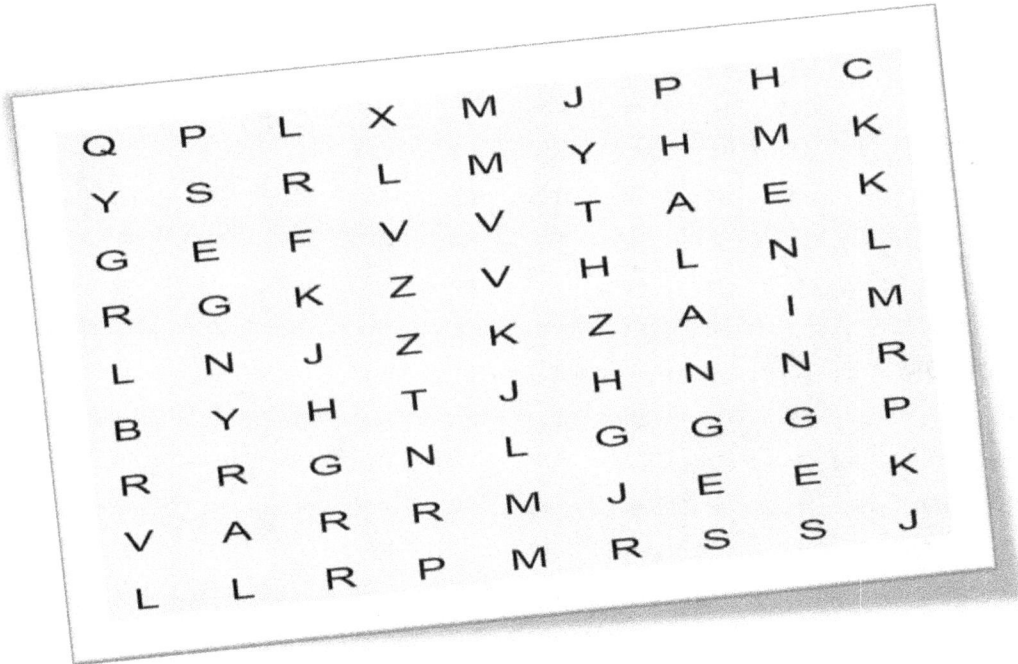

Plural nouns   **LOCATE ON THE GRID, THE SINGULAR FOR EACH LISTED PLURAL NOUN.**

LARYNGES

PHALANGES

MENINGES

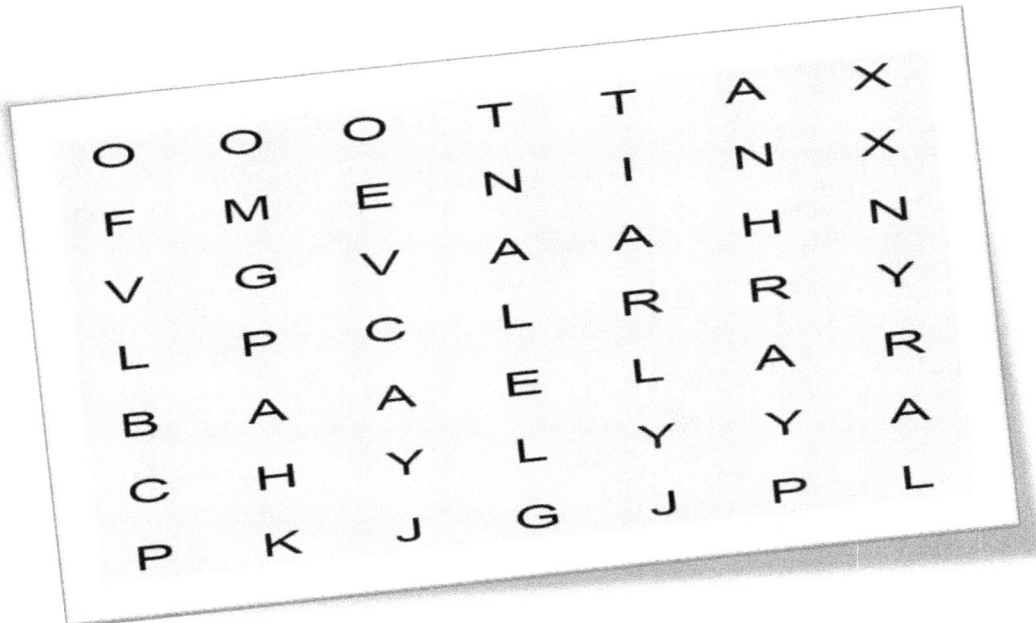

Give up? Solutions are on Pages 70 & 77.

Rule # 6. Some singular medical nouns that end with *um* are pluralized by dropping the endings and adding *a*.

Example: *um*   acetabul*um*   *a*   acetabul*a*

Singular nouns   **LOCATE ON THE GRID, THE PLURAL FOR EACH LISTED SINGULAR NOUN.**

SEPTUM

ANTRUM

ENDOCARDIUM

ATRIUM

BACTERIUM

ILEUM

OVUM

DIVERTICULUM

LABIUM

MEDIUM

ACETABULUM

MYOCARDIUM

D	H	Q	K	K	L	P	K	L	T	B	N
D	K	A	C	E	T	A	B	U	L	A	B
E	I	C	L	N	Q	L	N	D	R	V	G
N	A	V	N	B	A	C	T	E	R	I	A
D	I	I	E	M	N	W	G	F	L	Z	Q
O	D	N	D	R	V	X	G	E	A	A	F
C	R	B	N	E	T	R	A	I	X	R	X
A	A	K	Q	K	M	I	R	T	M	T	B
R	C	B	J	M	P	T	C	J	J	N	M
D	O	K	G	J	A	T	M	U	P	A	A
I	Y	A	I	B	A	L	V	H	L	V	L
A	M	W	X	S	E	P	T	A	O	A	Y

Plural nouns   **LOCATE ON THE GRID, THE SINGULAR FOR EACH LISTED PLURAL NOUN.**

ACETABULA

ANTRA

ATRIA

BACTERIA

DIVERTICULA

ENDOCARDIA

ILEA

LABIA

MEDIA

MYOCARDIA

OVA

SEPTA

L	A	N	E	N	D	O	C	A	R	D	I	U	M
Y	M	T	X	H	M	H	M	Y	C	L	N	I	N
J	U	D	R	J	N	U	M	K	X	G	L	T	M
B	L	R	K	I	R	L	I	D	B	E	M	L	U
A	U	P	R	T	U	D	T	B	U	L	D	Y	I
C	C	L	N	C	W	M	F	M	A	N	C	D	D
T	I	A	A	C	E	T	A	B	U	L	U	M	R
E	T	F	M	L	K	J	V	M	U	V	O	D	A
R	R	K	K	W	D	R	M	J	V	N	Q	L	C
I	E	T	K	H	D	U	U	N	M	C	W	P	O
U	V	T	T	X	I	P	T	C	K	P	N	G	Y
M	I	J	L	D	F	L	P	R	C	R	W	T	M
K	D	B	E	M	Y	V	E	R	G	G	Q	Y	W
B	V	M	Q	F	M	L	S	Y	C	N	Z	R	N

MEGA PUZZLE CLUE

The last unused letter on grid 7b is the Mega Puzzle letter for # 2, 7, 36, 40, 50, 62, 63, 71, 79, 111.

Give up? Solutions are on Pages 70 & 77

11

Rule # 7. Some singular medical nouns that end with *us* are pluralized by dropping the endings and adding *i*.
Example: *us*   calcul*us*   *i*   calcul*i*
Exceptions: Some singular medical nouns do not follow the "*us*" rule. Some of these include:

us	corp*us*	*ora*	corp*ora*
us	plex*us*	*es*	plexus*es*

LOCATE ON THE GRID, THE PLURAL FOR EACH LISTED SINGULAR NOUN.

Singular nouns
BRONCHUS
NUCLEUS
DIGITUS
COCCUS
CALCULUS
ESOPHAGUS
EMBOLUS
FUNGUS
MENISCUS
GLOMERULUS
EXCEPTIONS:
SINUS
CORPUS
PLEXUS
VIRUS
viscus

J	E	P	L	E	X	U	S	E	S	I	N
V	I	S	C	E	R	A	I	V	I	L	V
V	I	L	O	B	M	E	V	A	L	U	K
W	B	I	C	P	L	Y	R	B	U	C	K
J	R	N	G	C	H	O	R	C	R	L	W
V	O	R	U	N	P	A	O	K	E	A	M
M	N	N	R	R	U	C	G	P	M	C	E
J	C	T	O	T	C	F	N	I	O	R	N
Z	H	C	L	I	H	K	B	V	L	K	I
M	I	S	E	S	U	N	I	S	G	L	S
P	M	V	I	R	U	S	E	S	C	H	C
X	M	W	J	D	I	G	I	T	I	N	I

LOCATE ON THE GRID, THE SINGULAR FOR EACH LISTED PLURAL NOUN.

Plural nouns
CALCULI
NUCLEI
DIGITI
ESOPHAGI
BRONCHI
COCCI
EMBOLI
FUNGI
GLOMERULI
MENISCI
EXCEPTIONS:
CORPORA
PLEXUSES
SINUSES
VIRUSES
VISCERA

X	S	L	M	V	I	S	C	U	S	P	D
V	Y	U	K	Q	U	S	F	T	S	T	K
Y	C	J	N	E	C	U	C	R	U	C	S
C	J	R	L	I	N	H	O	C	C	T	U
C	O	C	N	G	S	C	R	A	S	Z	G
K	U	C	U	J	S	N	P	L	I	R	A
N	R	S	C	U	L	O	U	C	N	Q	H
C	M	T	X	U	Y	R	S	U	E	S	P
Q	G	E	F	T	S	B	Q	L	M	U	O
G	L	O	M	E	R	U	L	U	S	R	S
P	D	I	G	I	T	U	S	S	P	I	E
Q	C	K	S	U	L	O	B	M	E	V	B

MEGA PUZZLE CLUE
The last unused letter on grid 8a is the Mega Puzzle letter for # 113, 116, 123, 148, 161, 241, 244, 268, 270 & 331.

Give up? Solutions are on Pages 70 & 77

12

Rule # 8. Most singular medical nouns form their plural by adding _s_.
Example: _e_   bronchoscop_e_   _s_   bronchoscope_s_

Singular nouns   LOCATE ON THE GRID, THE PLURAL FOR EACH LISTED SINGULAR NOUN.

FINGER

BRONCHOSCOPE

VEIN

DISEASE

ENDOSCOPE

GLAND

TENDON

Plural nouns   LOCATE ON THE GRID, THE SINGULAR FOR EACH LISTED PLURAL NOUN.

BRONCHOSCOPES

DISEASES

ENDOSCOPES

FINGERS

GLANDS

TENDONS

VEINS

MEGA- PUZZLE CLUE
The last unused letter on grid 9a is the Mega Puzzle letter for # 1,
22, 54, 55, 140, 142, 150, 185, 189, 198.

Give up? Solutions are on Pages 70 & 77

13

Rules # 9. Some singular medical nouns form their plural by adding *ies*. If they end in y after a consonant.

Example: *y*   arter*y*   *ies*   arter*ies*

Singular nouns   *LOCATE ON THE GRID, THE PLURAL FOR EACH LISTED SINGULAR NOUN.*

CARDIOMYOPATHY

ARTERY

THERAPY

BRONCHOSCOPY

OVARY

BIOPSY

DEFORMITY

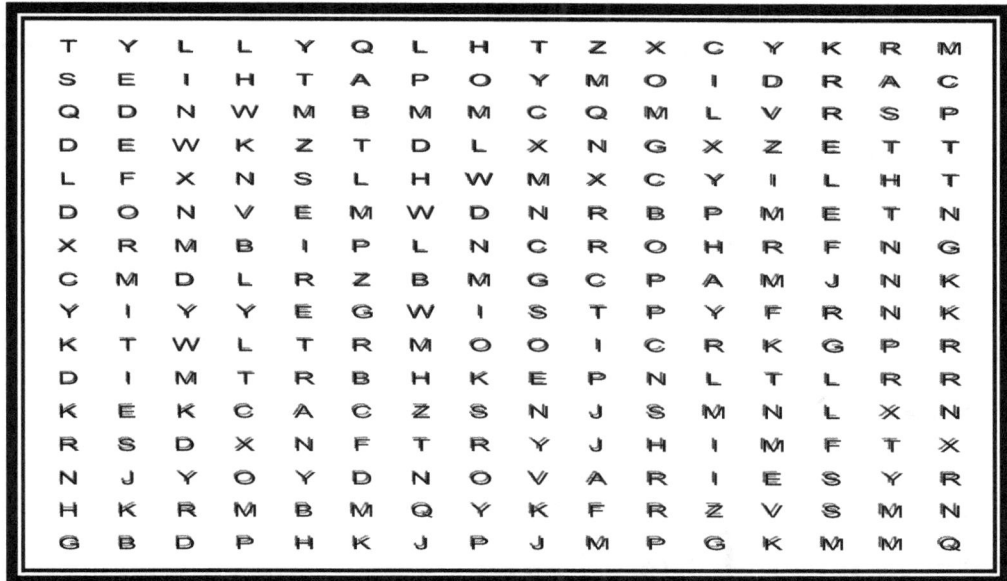

Plural nouns   *LOCATE ON THE GRID, THE SINGULAR FOR EACH LISTED PLURAL NOUN.*

ARTERIES

BRONCHOSCOPIES

OVARIES

BIOPSIES

DEFORMITIES

THERAPIES

CARDIOMYOPATHIES

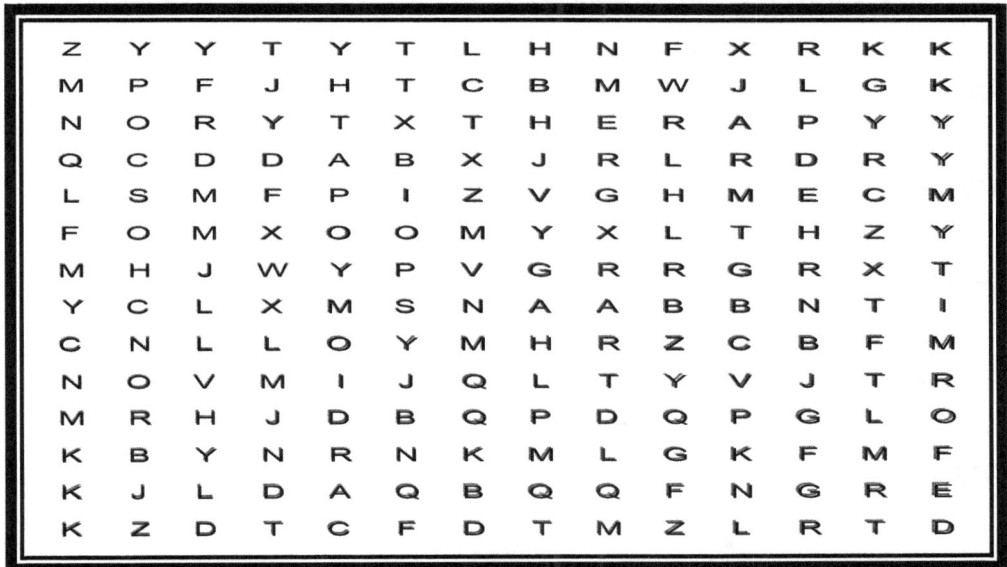

MEGA- PUZZLE CLUE
The last unused letter on grid 10b is the Mega Puzzle letter for # 11, 92, 108, 129, 145, 165, 172, 186, 209 & 238.

Give up? Solutions are on Pages 71 & 77

Rule # 10. Some singular nouns that end with *ch, sh, x, ss* or *s* are pluralized by dropping the endings and adding *es*.

Example: *ss*   absce*ss*   *es*   abscess*es*

LOCATE ON THE GRID, THE PLURAL FOR EACH LISTED SINGULAR NOUN.

Singular nouns

CRUTCH

ABSCESS

BYPASS

PATCH

H	T	A	K	B	T	P	B		L
S	F	B	S	L	H	D	R		Z
E	P	S	E	L	D	S	Z		Q
S	Q	C	H	L	L	E	H		Y
S	R	E	C	N	N	H	K		R
A	F	S	T	C	R	C	P		L
P	T	S	U	D	C	T	P		D
Y	M	E	R	L	H	A	Q		K
B	M	S	C	X	Y	P	L		F

LOCATE ON THE GRID, THE SINGULAR FOR EACH LISTED PLURAL NOUN.

Plural nouns

ABSCESSES

CRUTCHES

BYPASSES

PATCHES

I	G	E	T	S	M	A
H	C	T	A	P	A	B
C	B	Y	P	A	S	S
T	S	H	E	D	D	C
U	A	T	R	T	U	E
R	U	C	Y	R	R	S
C	I	L	H	A	K	S

Give up? Solutions are on Pages 71 & 77

15

Chapter 3

Adjectives and Root Words

Some medical words don't follow the normal rules in English to form their adjectives.
Example: heart   cardiac

ABDOMEN	ANTRUM	GONAD	HIATUS
BLADDER	APPENDIX	HYPOTHALAMUS	MAXILLA
*CECUM	ARM	MEDICINE	PENIS
DECIDUA	ARYEPIGLOTTICUS	MOUTH	PIA
EAR	ATRIUM	MANIA	PROSTATE
FACE	COMMISSURE	FOCUS	
GESTATION	EYE	ILEUM	
~~HEART~~	FIBULA	GYRUS	

LOCATE ON GRID, THE COMMON ADJECTIVE USED FOR EACH LISTED WORD.

```
C  A  A  L  A  N  O  I  T  A  T  S  E  G  C  R  C  M  C
G  L  A  R  Y  E  P  I  G  L  O  T  T  I  C  H  A  R  I
D  O  L  L  H  Y  A  A  A  E  R  T  R  L  I  S  S  S  M
P  P  L  A  A  D  B  R  A  C  H  I  A  L  H  E  P  N  A
T  T  A  N  D  N  T  A  C  L  A  E  L  I  A  G  R  C  L
Q  K  I  I  V  A  T  L  N  A  N  P  L  R  L  L  N  B  A
Z  T  R  M  L  Y  N  R  R  N  I  C  I  A  M  N  T  C  H
B  W  T  O  A  P  M  O  A  H  L  D  C  A  R  V  V  L  T
C  R  A  D  T  H  G  K  G  L  F  I  R  Z  L  Y  A  G  O
O  Q  L  B  A  X  C  J  W  A  S  Y  K  A  L  E  G  M  P
M  D  J  A  I  W  Z  R  C  E  R  C  F  A  C  T  L  A  Y
M  M  E  R  H  H  Q  I  V  A  K  O  C  I  G  H  K  N  H
I  K  C  C  H  C  A  K  L  J  C  I  D  F  O  M  L  I  C
S  M  Q  W  I  L  M  L  O  A  D  N  M  Q  C  R  F  C  A
S  T  C  Z  D  D  I  C  L  E  E  G  C  K  T  M  A  Q  U
U  Q  H  B  N  X  U  Z  M  P  D  V  C  E  C  A  L  L  R
R  L  W  K  A  L  K  A  P  P  N  R  A  L  U  B  I  F  A
A  F  Y  M  A  V  T  A  L  C  I  T  A  T  S  O  R  P  L
L  V  L  R  J  P  E  N  I  L  E  R  X  T  W  B  L  K  L
```

*

MEGA PUZZLE CLUE
The last unused letter on grid 12 is the Mega Puzzle letter for # 10, 27, 33,
90, 106, 128, 155, 183, 196 & 213.

Give up? Solutions are on Pages 71 & 78

FILL IN THE MISSING LETTERS FOR EACH LISTED ROOT WORD AND THEN LOCATE THEM ON THE GRID TO CHECK IF THEY ARE CORRECT. A N G I O IS DONE FOR YOU.

A̲ N̲ G̲I̲O̲-: RELATED TO BLOOD VESSELS

_ _ _ _ I̲-: OF OR PERTAINING TO THE HEART

_ _ _ _ R̲-: RELATED TO A JOINT

_ _ _ _ N̲ - OF OR RELATING TO ADRENAL GLANDS

_ _ _ _ O̲-: RELATED TO THE VAGINA

_ _ _ _ O̲ -: RELATED TO THE NOSE

_ _ _ _ O̲-: RELATED TO THE BLADDER

_ _ _ _ O̲ -: RELATED TO THE BREAST

_ _ _ _ R̲-: RELATED TO STOMACH

_ _ _ _ R̲ -: RELATED TO THE ABDOMINAL CAVITY

_ _ _ _ T̲ -: RELATED TO THE LIVER

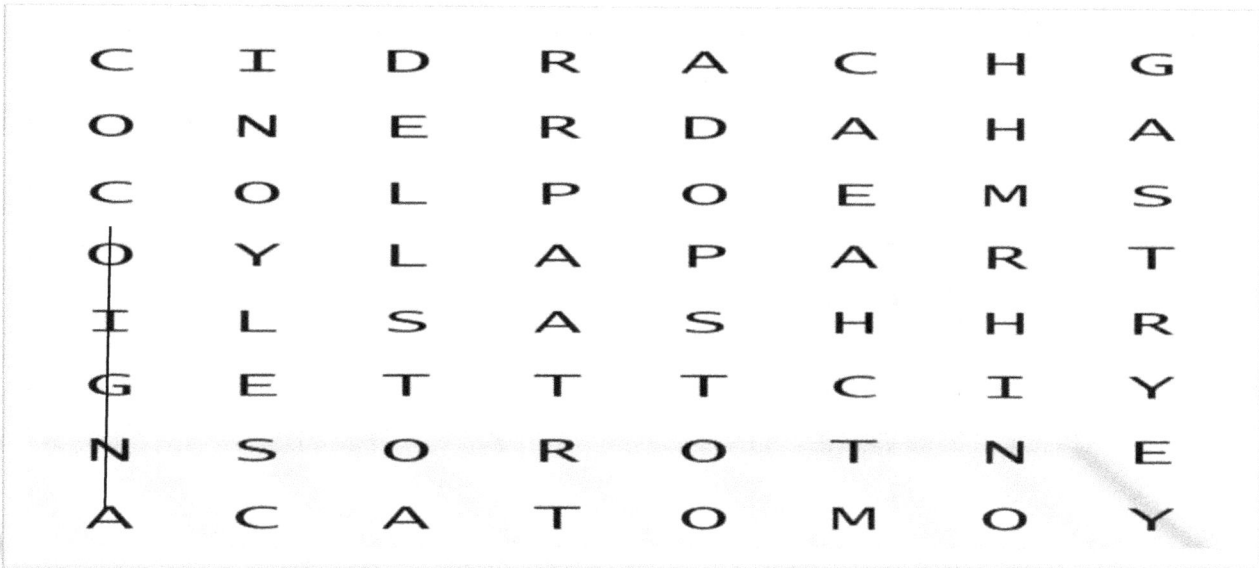

C	I	D	R	A	C	H	G
O	N	E	R	D	A	H	A
C	O	L	P	O	E	M	S
O	Y	L	A	P	A	R	T
I	L	S	A	S	H	H	R
G	E	T	T	T	C	I	Y
N	S	O	R	O	T	N	E
A	C	A	T	O	M	O	Y

BONUS

_ _ _ _ _ _ _ _ _ _ O̶ _ _ _ _

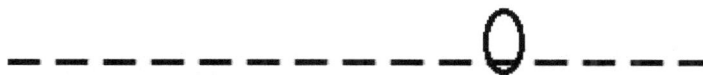

The first FIFTEEN unused letters on the grid reveal a word.

Need help? The first ten unused letters on puzzle # 12 grid are the first letters.
Need more help? The second set of the ten unused letters on puzzle # 12 grid are the second letters.
Need extra help? The third set of the ten unused letters on puzzle # 12 grid are the third letters.
Last help. The fourth set of the ten unused letters on puzzle # 12 grid are the fourth letters.

MEGA- PUZZLE CLUE

The letter that is circled in the bonus word is the mega puzzle letter for # 16, 20, 24, 29, 34, 38, 82, 88, 98 & 101.

Give up? Solutions are on Pages 71 & 79.

LOCATE ON THE GRID, THE COMMON ADJECTIVE USED FOR EACH LISTED WORD.

ANATOMY	**CUTIS**	**LARYNX**	**ISCHIUM**
BONE	**CYTOLOGY**	**LABIUM**	**GLUTEUS**
CEREBRUM	**ETHMOID**	**PELVIS**	**DURA**
DERMIS	**HYPOPHYSIS**	**OMENTUM**	**DUODENUM**
EMBRYO	**INTESTINE**	**GLOTTIS**	**UTERUS**
FASCIA	**MUCUS**	**MENINGES**	**URETER**
GINGIVA	**TRACHEA**	**METAPHYSIS**	
ARTERY	**THYMUS**	**RECTUM**	

```
T   A   C   S   U   O   E   S   S   O   L   A   R   E   T   E   R   U   G
O   H   E   M   B   R   Y   O   N   I   C   F   A   H   A   L   C   A   D
L   M   Y   L   A   E   S   Y   H   P   A   T   E   M   A   A   G   C   L
E   A   E   M   D   R   O   Y   A   D   P   E   L   V   I   C   E   N   A
H   N   R   I   C   T   E   M   E   O   A   I   I   S   N   C   E   R   R
M   G   I   B   T   C   L   E   O   O   M   G   N   L   N   G   N   L   Y
L   C   P   R   E   A   T   A   R   R   N   O   L   A   I   L   N   C   N
A   U   A   I   E   R   L   L   E   I   U   T   A   E   I   O   Y   U   G
I   T   P   R   K   T   E   D   G   S   A   Y   C   T   N   T   D   C   E
C   A   W   C   D   L   U   C   G   R   H   L   I   U   O   T   T   L   A
S   N   L   A   I   D   O   M   H   T   E   P   M   L   Q   I   L   A   L
A   E   K   F   R   L   L   D   F   L   X   E   O   G   R   C   L   N   W
F   O   R   C   M   A   W   A   A   H   N   G   T   P   R   Y   A   I   L
D   U   G   N   S   L   L   B   T   I   I   H   A   D   Y   F   I   T   K
D   S   D   O   A   T   I   Y   N   C   K   V   N   K   L   H   H   S   M
R   F   C   R   K   A   N   G   A   N   E   N   A   M   R   K   C   E   B
F   U   U   T   L   M   E   L   Q   T   X   R   T   W   L   R   S   T   R
M   D   R   Z   T   A   J   N   D   U   O   D   E   N   A   L   I   N   M
G   R   J   L   L   K   T   R   A   C   H   E   A   L   C   P   R   I   Z
```

Give up? Solutions are on Pages 71 & 78

FILL IN THE MISSING LETTERS FOR EACH LISTED ROOT WORD AND THEN LOCATE THEM ON THE
PUZZLE GRID TO CHECK IF THEY ARE CORRECT.

D	E	N	T	H	E	M	I
F	L	G	Y	N	O	N	T
G	A	O	O	R	M	S	U
P	E	C	H	A	O	R	O
I	A	N	I	C	H	H	C
D	D	O	U	E	I	D	A
A	E	E	M	I	G	N	A
C	N	A	P	L	O	C	T

_ _ _ _ _ (O)- OF OR RELATING TO FAT OR FATTY TISSUE

_ _ _ _ _ (O)- OF OR PERTAINING TO THE RIBS

_ _ _ _ _- PERTAINING TO FEMALE GENITAL

_ _ _ _ _- OF OR PERTAINING TO THE FACE

_ _ _ _ _- OF OR RELATING TO A GLAND

_ _ _ _ _- PERTAIN TO THE BLOOD

_ _ _ _ _ - PERTAINING TO BLOOD VESSEL

_ _ _ _ _ (E)- OF OR PERTAINING TO BILE

_ _ _ _ _- OF OR RELATING TO HEARING

_ _ _ _ _- OF OR PERTAINING TO TEETH

_ _ _ _ _- PERTAINING TO THE MEMBRANOUS FETAL SAC

_ _ _ _ _- OF OR PERTAINING TO THE KNEE

_ _ _ _ _ (O)- OF OR PERTAINING TO THE VAGINA

BONUS

_ _ _ _ _ _ _ _ _ _ _ _ _

The first THIRTEEN unused letters on the grid reveal a word.

MEGA- PUZZLE CLUE

The letter that is circled in the bonus word is the mega puzzle letter for # 104, 114, 118, 134, 138, 156, 159, 178, 203, 207.

Need help? The first thirteen unused letters on puzzle # 14 grid are the first letters.
Need more help? The second set of the thirteen unused letters on puzzle # 14 grid are the second letters.
Need extra help? The third set of the thirteen unused letters on puzzle # 14 grid are the third letters.
Last help. The fourth set of the thirteen unused letters on puzzle # 14 grid are the fourth letters.

Give up? Solutions are on Pages 71 & 79.

LOCATE ON THE GRID, THE COMMON ADJECTIVE USED FOR THE EACH LISTED WORD.

TONGUE	CLITORIS	ESOPHAGUS	VAGINA	DORSUM
OVARY	*FECES	*FOETUS	VEIN	COITUS
LETHARGY	GLAND	FOOT	ANUS	HERNIA
LEUKOCYTE	HEMIPLEGIA	ORBIT	AORTA	JEJUNUM
ADNEXA	CRANIUM	VIRUS	ALVEOLUS	SPINE
BRACHIUM	CUTICLE	VERTEBRA	BRONCHUS	SPLEEN

```
O  O  G  L  G  L  H  L  A  I  H  C  N  O  R  B  C  C
R  O  L  A  I  A  Y  Y  E  O  C  C  R  A  N  I  A  L
V  P  A  R  N  U  N  R  A  L  O  E  V  L  A  B  S  R
L  E  T  I  H  G  L  A  R  O  T  I  L  C  R  A  H  G
E  T  I  V  V  N  S  P  L  E  N  I  C  A  O  N  I  O
C  I  O  N  C  I  E  A  I  N  D  K  C  N  A  A  J  L
L  U  C  L  O  L  N  N  R  M  H  A  O  J  L  A  N
R  A  T  N  E  U  L  D  P  C  I  I  R  F  L  R  H  G
N  L  C  I  J  U  S  W  I  A  R  T  O  M  B  N  Z  E
G  P  A  E  C  T  K  G  L  A  I  E  M  E  A  T  R  S
H  T  J  S  F  U  E  O  V  C  T  W  T  M  D  Y  A  O
L  J  K  C  R  L  L  O  C  A  M  R  R  Y  N  Q  L  P
G  A  M  K  P  O  L  A  L  Y  E  K  T  J  E  S  U  H
R  L  T  I  J  L  D  J  R  V  T  B  Y  N  X  P  D  A
D  V  M  I  L  E  T  H  A  R  G  I  C  W  A  I  N  G
R  E  N  N  B  R  R  M  X  Z  L  T  C  V  L  N  A  E
H  L  A  I  N  R  E  H  X  L  A  D  E  P  Y  A  L  A
B  D  W  P  M  C  O  X  P  V  A  G  I  N  A  L  G  L
```

*Also spelled faeces.

*Also spelled fetus.

Give up? Solutions are on Pages 71 & 78.

FILL IN THE LETTERS FOR EACH LISTED ROOT WORD AND THEN LOCATE THEM ON THE PUZZLE GRID TO CHECK IF THEY ARE CORRECT.

_ _ _ _ _ D-: RELATED TO THE TESTICLE

_ _ _ _ _ R-: RELATED TO THE OVARY

_ _ _ _ _ V-: OF OR PERTAINING TO THE GUMS

_ _ _ _ _ O-: PERTAINING TO THE FEMALE GENITAL

_ _ _ _ _ R O: OF OR PERTAINING TO THE WOMB, THE UTERUS

_ _ _ _ _ C-: OF OR PERTAINING TO THE NECK

_ _ _ _ _ O-: RELATED TO LARGE INTESTINE COLON

BONUS

_ _ _ _ _ _ _ _ _ _ _ _ _

The first THIRTEEN unused letters on the grid reveal a word.

H	D	G	I	N	G	I	V
Y	I	O	N	O	L	O	C
S	H	G	P	R	R	O	C
T	C	S	Y	O	T	E	A
E	R	T	H	N	R	E	C
R	O	P	T	V	E	O	M
O	O	Y	I	T	X	C	M
O	X	C	W	P	Q	N	O

Need help? The first seven unused letters on puzzle # 16 grid are the first letters.

Need more help? The second set of the seven unused letters on puzzle # 16 grid are the second letters.

Need extra help? The third set of the seven unused letters on puzzle # 16 grid are the third letters.

MEGA- PUZZLE CLUE

The letter that is circled in the bonus word is the Mega Puzzle letter for # 5, 14, 47, 48, 73, 80, 96, 132, 146 & 163.

Give up? Solutions are on Pages 72 & 79.

Chapter 4

Detour

Sudoku Madness

Super Sudoku

4×4 blocks

Complete the grid so that every row, column and every four-by-four box contains all the digits 0 to 9 and the letters A to F. Solve the puzzle by logic and reasoning alone.

EVERY COLUMN AND ROW MUST ADD UP TO 45

					6				1						
4	E	9	8	5									7	6	1
5		D		3	0	F				7		4			
	2	3	7	1				E	4			C			
A	6									D		F			
	4				B		A			0					2
C	D			F	0			4	3			5			
	0	2			7				9			8	C		
				5			D					E			
B						1		3	9	A	6				F
				E		8			F	C		A	2		6
1			3	2	9	A					5		0		
					8			0				5	4		
E		B							1		7			9	8
	C	4			1	6		9				D			
	1	7		F	C							6	3	E	

Give up? Solutions are on Pages 72.

Sudoku

**The object is to place the numbers 1 to 9 in the empty squares so that each row, each column and each 3x3 box contains the same number only once.
EVERY COLUMN AND ROW MUST ADD UP TO 45.**

	9	8			2	1		
	3	5	1			6		
				8		7		
7		1	2		5			
9		4						8
6	4	7	3					5
			4				9	
				5		3		

Give up? Solutions are on Pages 72.

Letter Sudoku

Solve the puzzle the same way that you'd solve a numeric sudoku. Each of the letters A, B C, D, E, F, G, H, I, J, K, L M, N, O, P, Q, R, S, T, U, V, Q, X and Y is found once in every row, column and 5×5 box.

Give up? Solutions are on Pages 72.

Letter Sudoku

Solve the puzzle the same way that you'd solve a numeric sudoku. Each of the letters A, B, C, D, E, F, G, H, I, J, K, L, M, N, O, P, Q, R, S, T, U, V, Q, X and Y is found once in every row, column and 5×5 box.

S	O		E		Q		I									Y	D		H			U		
	F	C	B	K	X			L					O		V	W							J	
T			D	J	F			N	B	A	H		K				G		R				L	
L		W		P		D		O	C		U					S	M				E			
			M		W						G						E							
J	W	N			Y		U	M		X	L	P				F		T					A	O
	H			E			W	C	F	M		I		P		X	Y			N				
	D	A							G	T			W	H	U					Q		M		
		F		O			I			W		H		N		A	S	P	E	J				
O		Y	I			S	H	J		R	D	C			L	V	Q			T	X			
		L			I		C			R	Q		U	P		B					T	E		
M			H	V		L			K	O	N	B	S	I		R			G					
N	E		Y			R			A	F		H	M	C							B			
R			U	K	J		M	V		S	I			D	L		Q		F					
U			D					J	Y	E		F		A		N	S		R					
P	C		U		L			N	F		T				D		X		O	V				
	T	W	A	B				E		J					X		K		Y					
Y		F		A	E	U	D		Q		K			G					B					
L		Q		T	H		V		O				P		D	M	J	U						
H		B		F	P	S	Y	U		W		L	T		A									
	V	J	L		B	S	K		O		Y	F	A	E				G	W					
G		D	L		Y	M		E	T		H		X				C	S	A					
		M			F			Q	X		D	N			Y	B	H	T						
E	Q	O				D	N	V	U						K									
	X	G		R			S		W	K	Q				P	L	F							

CHAPTER 5

MNEMONICS

Mnemonics are important to aid students and doctors remember the large amount of information in the field of medicine. Below is one of the mnemonics used to remember the cranial nerves.

"Ooh, Ooh, Ooh To Touch And Feel Very Good Velvet Such Heaven"

FILL THE BLANK SPACES FOR THE NAMES OF THE CRANIAL NERVES AND THEN LOCATE THEM ON THE GRID TO CHECK IF THEY ARE CORRECT.

Cranial nerves

CN 1 _ _ _ _ _ _ _ _ _

Cn2 _ _ _ _ _

Cn 3 _ _ _ _ _ _ _ _ _ _

Cn 4 _ _ _ _ _ _ _ _

Cn5 _ _ _ _ _ _ _ _ _

Cn 6 _ _ _ _ _ _ _

Cn 7 _ _ _ _ _ _

Cn 8 _ _ _ _ _ _ _ _

_ _ _ _ _ _ _ _ _

Cn 9 _ _ _ _ _ _ _ _

_ _ _ _ _ _ _ _

Cn 10 _ _ _ _ _

Cn11 _ _ _ _ _ _ _ _ _

Cn12 _ _ _ _ _ _ _ _ _ _ _ _

```
N L Q T L A I C A F L K C J Z B R
L K B N V J M K K S K I X M W J A
H A N R T X K Q U L T V C K L C E
D T E T T G P G T P C L T G B C L
Q Z K G W X A L O K L D R Y H V H
N P R J N V X Y K A M A I R J F C
T T Z W T Y T K S V B M G O J V O
W D R X Y R R S K D D C E T H M C
X Q G K H M O A U R Y B M C W N O
R M X V H L K C H P H G I A Z V L
V J P Q G R E N H P T Q N F R C U
W T K O G N B R T L O L A L P X B
T Z P D S N W C Q K E S L O T V I
F Y A C C E S S O R Y A S T M L T
H B K C G K L M N Z K B R O J T S
Q L T M R N G B L R P N M J L Z E
Z C T O C U L O M O T O R W Z G V
```

Need help? The first twelve unused letters on puzzle # 6b grid are the first letters for the listed twelve-cranial nerves.

Need more help? The second set of the twelve unused letters on puzzle # 6b grid are the second letters for the listed twelve-cranial nerves.

MEGA- PUZZLE CLUE
The last letter of the 9th CN is the Mega Puzzle letter for # 231, 246, 250, 254, 263, 279, 293, 316 & 329.

Give up? Solution is on Page 72.

Pancreatitis is an inflammatory process that occurs in the pancreas. It can be an acute (short-term) or chronic (long-term) condition. A commonly used mnemonic for the causes of pancreatitis is:

I GET SMASHED.

FILL THE BLANK SPACES FOR THE CAUSES OF PANCREATITIS AND THEN LOCATE THEM OF THE GRID TO CHECK IF THEY ARE CORRECT.

Causes of pancreatitis

1. _ _ _ _ _ _ _ _ _ _

2. _ _ _ _ _ _ _ _ _ _

3. _ _ _ _ _ _ _

4. _ _ _ _ _ _

5. _ _ _ _ _ _ _

6. _ _ _ _ _ / Malignancy

7. _ _ _ _ _ _ _ _ _ _

8. _ _ _ _ _ _ _ _

9*. _ _ _ _ _ _ _ _ _ _ _ _ _

/ Hypertriglycerides

10. _ _ _ _

11. _ _ _ _ _

P	L	B	H	H	Q	T	T	W	N	R	S	M	H
B	R	R	L	M	T	J	V	O	M	E	S	G	Y
E	T	H	A	N	O	L	I	U	N	X	T	B	P
K	P	M	M	L	T	P	M	O	L	W	E	C	E
N	J	L	N	M	R	P	T	C	M	L	R	V	R
D	K	H	N	O	S	S	C	I	J	M	O	H	C
F	L	M	C	R	L	T	G	H	V	C	I	H	A
M	L	S	J	L	P	D	R	T	W	R	D	H	L
L	P	K	A	R	L	V	Y	A	P	K	S	L	C
Z	S	G	N	R	F	L	W	P	U	C	L	T	A
G	G	M	R	X	M	L	D	O	D	M	R	T	E
H	U	Z	N	F	X	Y	R	I	N	N	A	E	M
Q	R	W	L	K	Z	K	G	D	D	D	V	J	I
B	D	Y	E	N	U	M	M	I	O	T	U	A	A

Need help? The first eleven unused letters on puzzle # 11b grid are the first letters for listed causes of pancreatitis. Need more help? The second set of the eleven unused letters on puzzle # 11b grid are the second letters for the listed causes of pancreatitis.

* Also spelled hypercalcemia.
Give up? Solution is on Page 72

MEGA- PUZZLE CLUE
The last letter of # 10 answer is the Mega Puzzle letter for # 205, 224, 233, 252, 274, 289, 318 & 325.

The Carpal bones are eight small bones that make up the wrist. The mnemonic Some Lovers Try Positions That They Cannot Handle is used to remember these small bones.

FILL THE BLANK SPACES FOR THE NAMES OF THE CARPAL BONES AND THEN LOCATE THEM ON THE PUZZLE GRID TO CHECK IF THEY ARE CORRECT.

The carpal bones are listed in alphabetical order.

1 _ _ _ _ _ _ _ _

2 _ _ _ _ _ _

3 _ _ _ _ _ _

4 _ _ _ _ _ _ _

5 _ _ _ _ _ _ _ _

6 _ _ _ _ _ _ _ _

7 _ _ _ _ _ _ _ _ _

8 _ _ _ _ _ _ _ _

X	T	R	A	P	E	Z	I	U	M	P
M	U	R	T	E	U	Q	I	R	T	E
S	E	P	T	G	K	F	F	L	T	T
C	T	M	I	J	G	J	Q	A	X	R
A	A	Q	C	S	D	D	M	B	R	A
P	T	H	Q	W	I	A	V	Z	R	P
H	I	N	C	K	H	F	M	Q	Q	E
O	P	F	M	T	T	G	O	V	N	Z
I	A	F	W	F	Q	B	M	R	F	O
D	C	B	K	K	K	L	R	C	M	I
C	L	U	N	A	T	E	B	K	W	D

Need help? The first eight unused letters on puzzle # 3b grid are the first letters for the listed eight-carpal bones. Need more help? The second set of the eight unused letters on puzzle # 3b grid are the second letters for the listed eight-carpal bones.

Give up? Solution is on Page 72.

Chapter 6

Abbreviations

To solve this puzzle, use unbroken lines in which the last letter of one abbreviation is the first letter of the next. Find your way through the puzzle to the finish. To get you started, NSTEMI has been marked as the starting. Use the listed abbreviations to aid your path by predicting the number of letters in the next abbreviation.

FIND YOUR WAY THROUGH MEDICAL SCHOOL!

N	S	T	E	M	I	X	C	V	Q	U	O	H	C	W
M	N	B	V	X	R	A	Z	Z	S	S	I	U	C	D
Q	W	E	R	T	D	Y	U	I	O	P	R	M	M	H
X	I	M	E	T	S	X	D	X	S	X	S	E	W	E
Q	U	D	F	F	G	P	C	C	F	G	S	G	Q	W
A	G	S	D	D	O	F	I	L	P	D	M	M	N	Q
A	R	O	S	C	Q	W	S	R	I	Y	U	I	O	L
A	S	D	C	D	F	I	E	S	D	F	G	H	H	K
S	D	F	E	E	R	E	R	E	L	E	R	E	R	W
A	S	R	A	S	I	A	D	H	D	C	D	D	F	C
C	S	F	D	O	Q	W	E	E	E	R	A	C	V	T
X	S	B	N	C	W	E	R	L	C	E	S	C	V	X
D	S	O	A	P	D	D	D	L	Q	Q	R	Q	W	E
S	D	F	G	H	J	J	K	P	R	O	M	A	S	D
A	S	D	D	D	D	D	D	F	F	F	F	F	F	Q

1. ▸ START N S T E M I

2. _ _ _ _
3. _ _ _ _ _
4. _ _ _ _
5. _ _ _ _
6. _ _ _ _
7. _ _ _ _

8. _ _ _ _
9. _ _ _ _
10. _ _ _ _
11. _ _ _ _
12. _ _ _ _
13. _ _ _ _ _
14. _ _ _ _ _
15. _ _ _ _

16. _ _ _ _
17. _ _ _ _
18. _ _ _ _
19. _ _ _ _

20. ◂ finish _ _ _ _

MEGA- PUZZLE CLUE
The first letter of the 10th abbreviation is the letter for the Mega Puzzle # 19, 25,43,45,52,58,59,72,75,76,87 & 117.

Give up? Solutions are on Pages 72 & 79.

Solve the puzzle by forming unbroken lines in which the last letter of one abbreviation is the first letter of the next abbreviation. Find your way through the puzzle to the finish. To get you started, NSTEMI has been marked as the starting.

FIND YOUR WAY THROUGH INTERNSHIP!

Q	W	C	I	U	G	R	Q	Z	D	M	A	R	D	finish
W	Z	V	M	A	A	O	W	X	L	I	Q	S	A	
E	X	B	E	S	S	E	C	K	A	C	D	S		
R	C	N	T	D	D	C	R	B	S	S	E	S	D	
T	V	N	S	F	F	D	A	L	Q	I	W	S	F	
Y	B	H	Q	O	G	F	C	B	W	D	R	S	G	
U	N	H	W	D	C	A	B	A	G	F	R	S	H	
I	M	D	E	F	F	P	A	O	S	G	T	F	D	
I	N	A	A	L	G	G	T	P	E	D	Y	G	F	
O	B	I	S	G	L	H	Y	O	R	F	I	J	G	
P	V	S	I	C	D	P	U	I	A	G	T	S	H	
L	C	Q	D	D	C	R	I	S	I	H	R	J	H	
J	F	W	F	D	U	O	R	I	D	A	T	H	J	
START	N	S	T	E	M	I	M	P	U	S	J	Y	G	O

1. START <u>N S T E M I</u>

2. _ _ _ _

3. _ _ _ _

4. _ _ _ _ _

5. _ _ _ _ _

6. _ _ _ _

7. _ _ _ _

8. _ _ _ _

9. _ _ _ _

10. _ _ _ _

11. _ _ _ _

12. _ _ _ _

13. _ _ _ _ _

14. _ _ _ _

15. _ _ _ _

16. _ _ _ _

17. _ _ _ _

18. _ _ _ _

19. _ _ _ _

20. _ _ _ _

21. _ _ _ _

22. _ _ _ _ _

MEGA- PUZZLE CLUE

The second letter of #11 abbreviation is the letter for the Mega Puzzle # 110, 139, 143, 149, 162, 166, 170 & 174.

Give up? Solutions are on Pages 73&79.

Solve the puzzle by forming unbroken lines in which the last letter of one abbreviation CAN BE THE FIRST or LAST letter of the next abbreviation. Find your way through the puzzle to the finish. To get you started, NSTEMI has been marked as the starting.

FIND YOUR WAY THROUGH POSTGRAD!

Q	W	C	I	U	G	R	Q	Z	D	M	A	R	D
W	Z	V	M	A	A	O	W	X	L	I	Q	S	A
E	X	B	E	S	S	E	C	K	A	C	D	S	
R	C	N	T	D	D	C	R	B	S	S	E	S	D
T	V	N	S	F	F	D	A	L	Q	I	W	S	F
Y	B	H	Q	O	G	F	C	B	W	D	R	S	G
U	N	H	W	D	C	A	B	A	G	F	R	S	H
I	M	D	E	F	F	P	A	O	S	G	T	F	D
I	N	A	A	L	G	G	T	P	E	D	Y	G	F
O	B	I	S	G	L	H	Y	O	R	F	I	J	G
P	V	S	I	C	D	P	U	I	A	G	T	S	H
L	C	Q	D	D	C	R	I	S	I	H	R	J	H
J	F	W	F	D	U	O	R	I	D	A	T	H	J
N	S	T	E	M	I	M	P	U	S	J	Y	G	O

1. N S T E M I	10. _ _ _ _	19. _ _ _ _
2. I R S S	11. _ _ _ _ *	20. _ _ _ _
3. _ _ _ _ _	12. _ _ _ _ _	21. _ _ _ _
4. _ _ _ _	13. _ _ _ _	22. _ _ _ _
5. _ _ _ _	14. _ _ _ _ *	23. _ _ _ _
6. _ _ _ _	15. _ _ _ _ _	24. _ _ _ _ _
7. _ _ _ _ *	16. _ _ _ _ _	25. D I C
8. _ _ _ _	17. _ _ _ _	
9. _ _ _ _	18. _ _ _ _	

Mega- puzzle clue
The first letter of the 9th abbreviation is the letter for the
Mega Puzzle # 144,153,167,169,171,175,182 & 188.

Give up? Solutions are on Pages 73 & 79.

CHAPTER 7

NINE & FIVE LETTER WORDS

To solve this puzzle, find the 15 nine-letter words in the shape of a G. The first letter of the word is given as a clue and is also center letter when located on the grid. The rest of the letters can be read clockwise or anticlockwise on the grid. Examples: PATHOLOGY is G as an example; notice the P is the first letter and the center letter on the grid.

P A T H O L O G Y   D _ _ _ _ _ _ _ _   A _ _ _ _ _ _ _ _

S _ _ _ _ _ _ _ _   N _ _ _ _ _ _ _ _   A _ _ _ _ _ _ _ _

H _ _ _ _ _ _ _ _   A _ _ _ _ _ _ _ _   P _ _ _ _ _ _ _ _

D _ _ _ _ _ _ _ _   V _ _ _ _ _ _ _ _   P _ _ _ _ _ _ _ _

H _ _ _ _ _ _ _ _   M _ _ _ _ _ _ _ _   P _ _ _ _ _ _ _ _

Y	A	T	F	A	N	E	Y	U	L	E	R	E	W	D
G	P	H	G	I	P	U	R	P	M	R	P	M	E	S
O	L	O	H	N	O	M	A	N	O	U	T	A	R	D
M	W	E	J	G	E	R	T	Y	L	S	S	E	M	Q
L	Q	W	E	F	D	D	B	N	D	D	E	M	B	W
O	G	S	D	D	F	U	A	O	A	U	N	A	R	E
I	F	D	D	R	D	C	T	I	T	C	A	A	R	R
U	D	S	D	E	S	R	T	R	O	T	L	V	I	T
E	A	I	A	R	I	A	H	E	S	O	L	E	C	Y
S	E	D	R	T	T	I	R	N	I	N	D	S	I	A
D	O	H	R	H	I	N	H	S	S	E	M	I	D	G
F	N	N	H	H	S	E	P	D	I	H	O	S	O	N
Q	O	I	I	F	N	N	F	E	S	Y	L	S	E	P
W	T	I	B	F	O	I	E	F	F	G	S	I	H	A
W	E	R	T	G	I	T	C	G	G	F	D	T	I	T

Give up? Solution is on Page 73.

Scan the grid in all directions for eleven pairs of 5- letter words. Each word in a pair crosses its partner through the center letter. They either form a "+" or an "x" shape. One pair is done to start you off.

<u>CHEST</u> X **<u>CLEFT.</u>**

------------ X/+ ------------,	------------ X/+ ------------,
------------ X/+ ------------,	------------ X/+ ------------,
------------ X/+ ------------,	------------ X/+ ------------,
----------- X/+ ------------,	------------ X/+ ------------,
----------- X/+ ------------,	------------ X/+ ------------

T	W	E	R	I	L	U	I	O	M	B	P	L	K	S
F	E	G	L	B	N	Y	D	U	F	G	L	H	T	J
F	G	E	G	Z	X	C	M	V	B	N	M	O	K	L
K	U	J	T	H	A	P	G	P	B	F	M	G	O	L
M	A	S	S	H	S	T	S	U	H	A	D	F	G	D
C	Z	X	C	S	V	B	R	M	N	P	J	P	L	S
A	R	S	H	D	F	S	G	I	H	J	E	I	I	K
Q	W	O	V	E	A	R	L	T	A	R	A	N	L	U
T	C	Y	U	A	U	A	I	O	P	L	U	N	I	K
K	J	H	G	P	R	F	D	S	A	S	Z	A	X	S
C	C	P	V	T	B	I	N	M	M	C	L	H	K	C
P	O	O	A	O	I	U	X	A	Y	T	H	R	L	E
P	O	L	I	O	A	M	A	N	I	A	D	X	F	H
H	U	Y	O	G	H	J	K	I	K	L	F	L	S	J
S	J	S	K	N	J	K	J	C	K	T	J	K	J	T

Give up? Solution is on Page 73.

Chapter 8

Pathognomonic Signs and Tests

Pathognomonic signs and tests are important in medicine because they indicate that a disease or condition is present beyond a doubt.

ACROSS

3. RIGLER'S SIGN
4. KOCHER'S SIGN & VON GRAEFE'S SIGN
6. WHIPPLE'S TRIAD
8. CHADWICK'S SIGN & GOODELL'S SIGN
9. HUTCHINSON'S FRECKLE
14. TROUSSEAU'S SIGN & CHVOSTEK'S SIGN
16. HUTCHINSON'S SIGN
20. BLUMBERG SIGN
21. KERNIG'S & BRUDZINSKI'S SIGN

22. HATCHCOCK'S SIGN
23. LARREY'S SIGN
25. PERICARDIAL FRICTION RUB
27. WINTERBOTTOM'S SIGN
28. TRAUBE'S SIGN

DOWN

1. GOTTRON'S PAPULES
2. *PILL-ROLLING TREMORS & MYERSON'S SIGN
5. KOEPPE'S NODULES
7. BOUCHARD'S & HEBERDEN'S NODE

10. MCBURNEY'S TENDERNESS & ROSENSTEIN'S SIGN
11. PSEUDOMEMBRANE ON TONSILS & PHARYNX
12. GUNN'S SIGN & SALUS'S SIGN
13. KVEIM TEST
15. KOPLIK'S SPOTS
17. BECHTEREW'S TEST
18. MURPHY'S SIGN
19. RICE-WATERY STOOL
24. TOPHI
26. LEVINE'S SIGN

ENTER ON THE GRID, THE DISEASE FOR EACH LISTED PATHOGNOMONIC SIGN OR TEST ACCORDING TO THEIR CORRESPONDING NUMBER.

MEGA- PUZZLE CLUE
The first letter of # 10 answer is the letter for the Mega Puzzle # 181, 197, 199, 221, 243, 245, 267, 278, 283, 287, 309, 315 & 319.

*Apostrophe "s" is not found on the grid.
Give up? Solution is on Page 73.

40

Chapter 9

Antidotes & Poisons

An antidote is a substance that counteracts a poison. A substance that can cause the illness or death of living organism when introduced or absorbed is called a poison.

ACROSS

1. METHYLENE BLUE
8. PRALIDOXIME CHLORIDE & ATROPINE
10. FLUMAZENIL
12. SUCCIMER
14. LEUCOVORIN
16. DIGOXIN IMMUNE FAB ANTIBODY

17. PYRIDOXINE
18. HYDROXOCOBALAMIN, AMYL NITRITE, SODIUM NITRITE, OR THIOSULFATE

DOWN

2. ETHANOL OR FOMEPIZOLE
3. N-ACETYLCYSTEINE
4. GLUCOSE

5. PRUSSIAN BLUE
6. DEFEROXAMINE MESYLATE
7. OCTREOTIDE ACETATE
9. PROTAMINE SULFATE
11. PHYTOMENADIONE (VITAMIN K) AND FRESH FROZEN PLASMA
13. THEOPHYLLINE
15. NALOXONE HYDROCHLORIDE

ENTER ON THE GRID THE POISON FOR EACH LISTED ANTIDOTE ACCORDING TO THEIR CORESPONDING NUMBER.

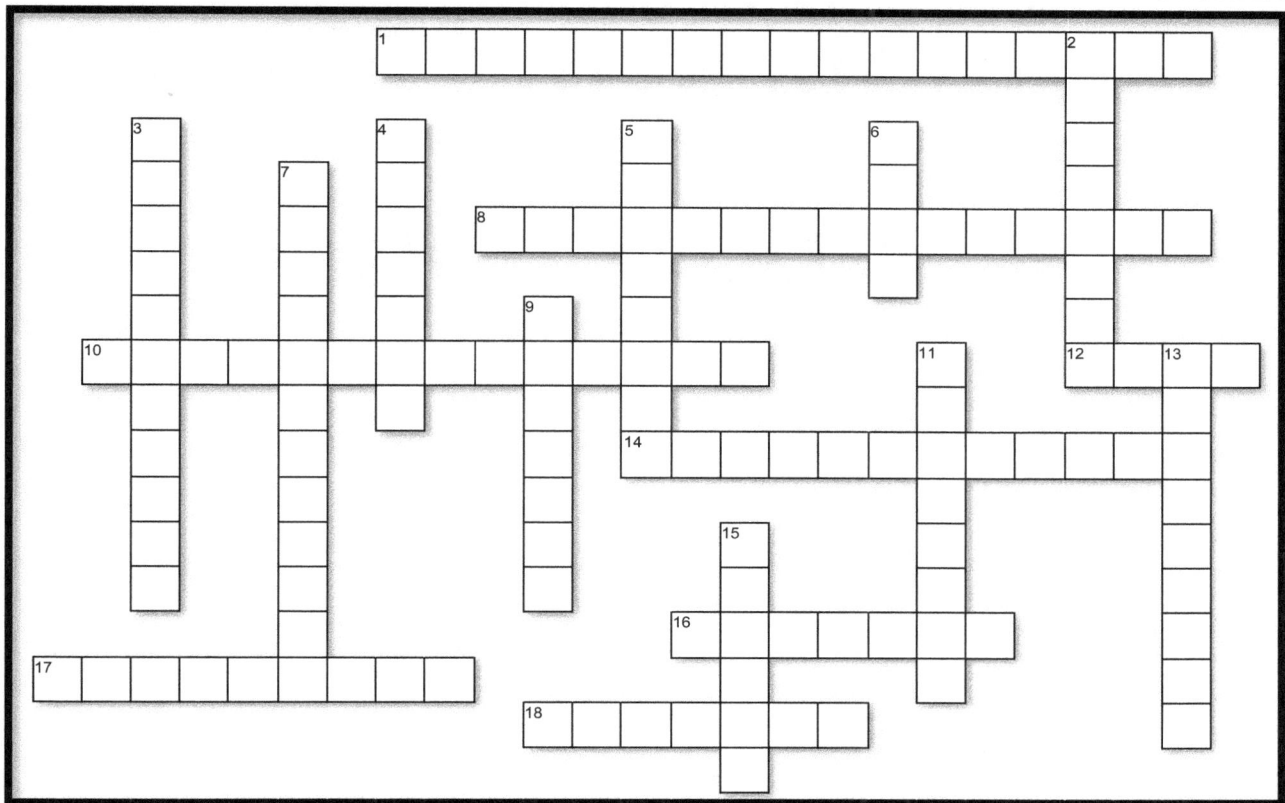

MEGA PUZZLE CLUE
The first letter of # 18 answer is the letter for the Mega Puzzle # 212, 237, 242, 248, 265, 271, 281, 286, 291, 297, 302 & 327.

Give up? Solution is on Page 73.

Chapter 10

Hormones and Site of Production

ACROSS

5. GASTRIN

7. ERYTHROPOIETIN

8. INSULIN

9. LH & OXYTOCIN

12. CALCITONIN

13. CHOLECYSTOKININ

DOWN

1. TESTOSTERONE

2. PROGESTERONE

3. ANP

4. VITAMIN D

6. TRH

10 ADRENALINE

11 T3 & T4

ENTER ON THE GRID THE SITE OF PRODUCTION FOR EACH LISTED HORMONE

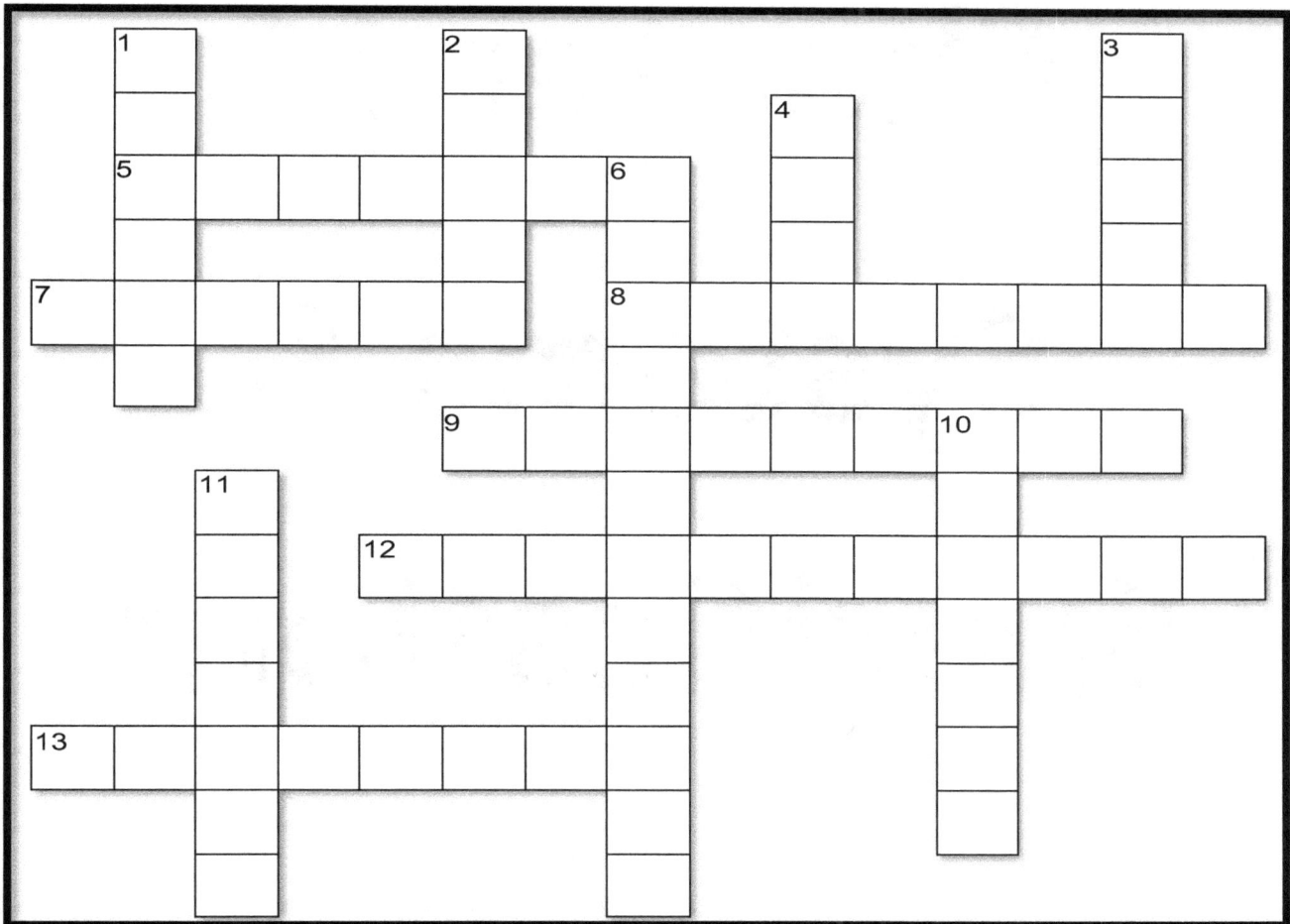

MEGA PUZZLE CLUE

The first letter of # 4 answer is the letter for the Mega Puzzle # 193, 195, 202, 211, 217, 219, 222, 227, 228, 261 & 280.

Give up? Solution is on Page 73.

Chapter 11

Systems & Specifications

ACROSS

2. RETURNS FLUID TO BLOOD & DEFENDS AGAINST PATHOGENS.

4. REMOVES CARBON DIOXIDE FROM THE BLOOD & DELIVERS OXYGEN TO THE BODY.

7. SUPPORTS THE BODY & ENABLES MOVEMENT.

8. ABSORBS NUTRIENTS AND EXCRETES WASTES.

9. DELIVERS OXYGEN AND NUTRIENTS TO TISSUES.

10. SECRETES HORMONES & REGULATES BODILY PROCESSES.

11. ENCLOSES INTERNAL BODY STRUCTURES & SITE OF MANY SENSORY RECEPTORS.

DOWN

1. DETECTS & PROCESSES SENSORY INFORMATION & CONTROL BODILY MOVEMENT.

3. ENABLES MOVEMENT & HELPS MAINTAIN BODY TEMPERATURE.

5. PRODUCES SEX HORMONES & PRODUCES MILK.

6 REMOVES & EXCRETES WASTE FROM THE BLOOD

ENTER ON THE GRID THE SYSTEM FOR EACH LISTED SPECIFICATION ACCORDING TO THEIR CORRESPONDING NUMBER

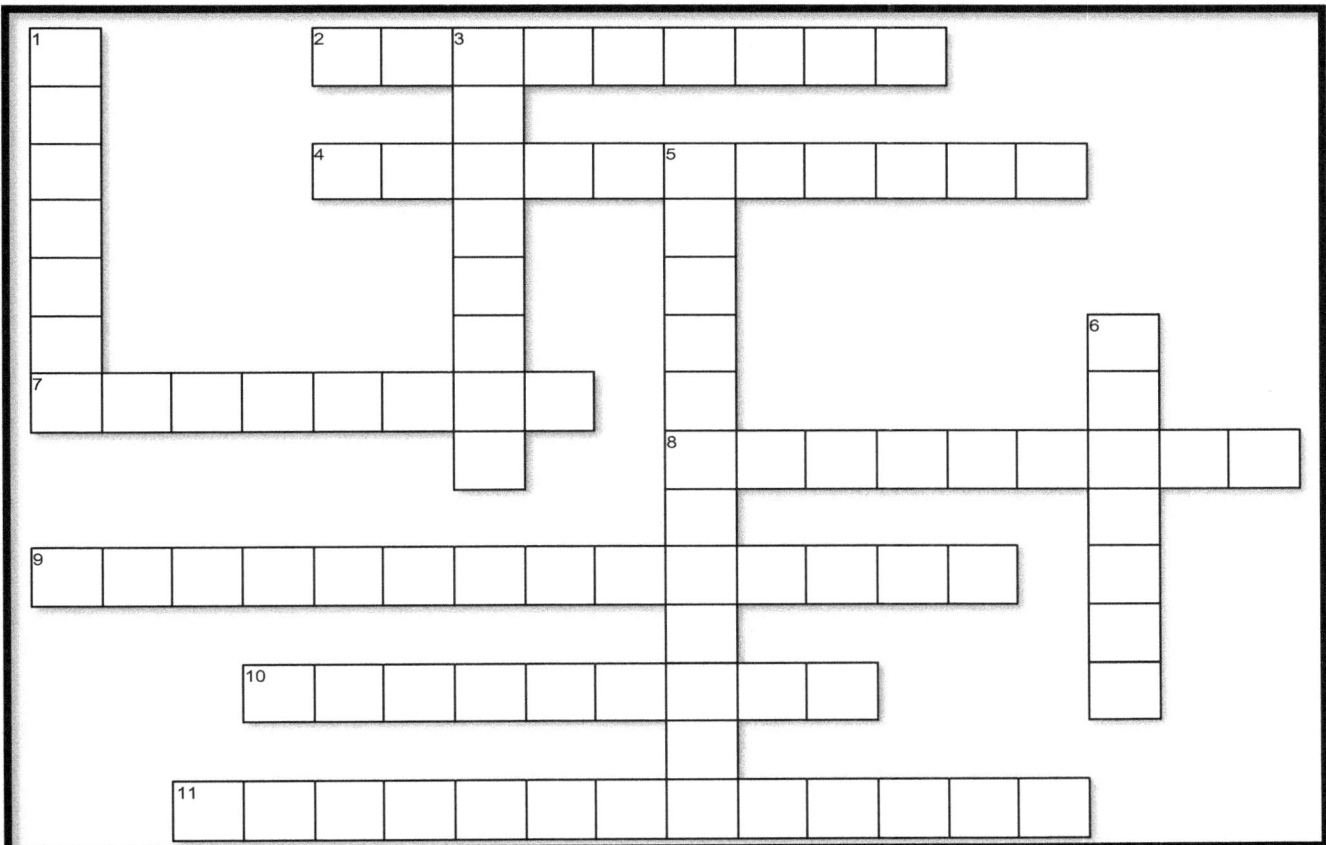

MEGA- PUZZLE CLUE

The first letter of # 6 answer is the letter for the Mega Puzzle # 9, 49, 53, 65, 89, 93, 105, 112, 121, 127 & 152.

Give up? Solution is on Page 73.

Chapter 12

Word Play

ENTER ON THE GRID, THE MEDICAL WORD THAT CAN BE FORMED BY ADDING OR SUBTRACTING A LETTER FROM EACH LISTED NON-MEDICAL WORD.

Example: KNEEL (NON-MEDICAL WORD): K N E E (MEDICAL WORD)

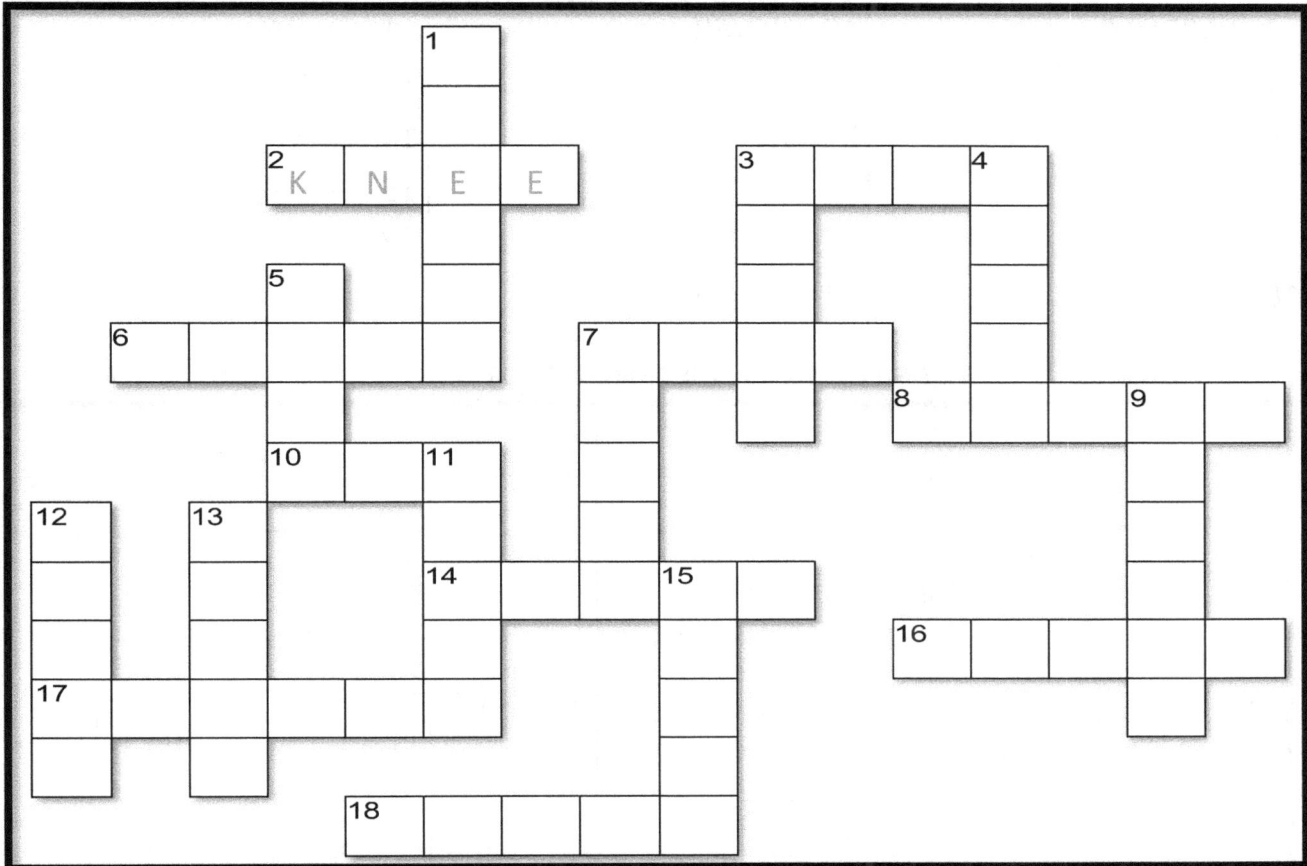

ACROSS

2. ~~KNEEL~~ K N E E

3. SKINK

6. HEAR

7. LUNGE

8. TEBETH

10. CRIB

14. LATRIA

16. PENS

17. TENON

18. SINS

DOWN

1. BEAST

3. SPIN

4. NERVED

5. AIR

7. SLIVER

9. TESTS

11. BRAN

12. MOUTHY

13. JOIN

15. INCUSE

MEGA- PUZZLE CLUE

The first letter of # 15 answer is the Mega Puzzle letter for # 218, 232, 239, 247, 251, 255, 258, 282, 285, 296, 301 & 317.

Give up? Solutions are on Pages 73 & 79.

An anagram is a meaningful word made after rearranging all the letters of a word.

ACROSS

3. LABRUM
4. HADE
5. PINES
7. INKS
8. EBON
10. RASCAL

12. VILER
16. EARTH
18. NEVER

DOWN

1. SUTRAS
2. RETAIN

6. DONE
9. BELOW
11. TIARA
13. VINE
14. HIGHT
15. SUTURE
17. KEEN

ENTER ON THE GRID, THE MEDICAL WORD (THE ANAGRAM) FOR EACH LISTED NON-MEDICAL WORD.

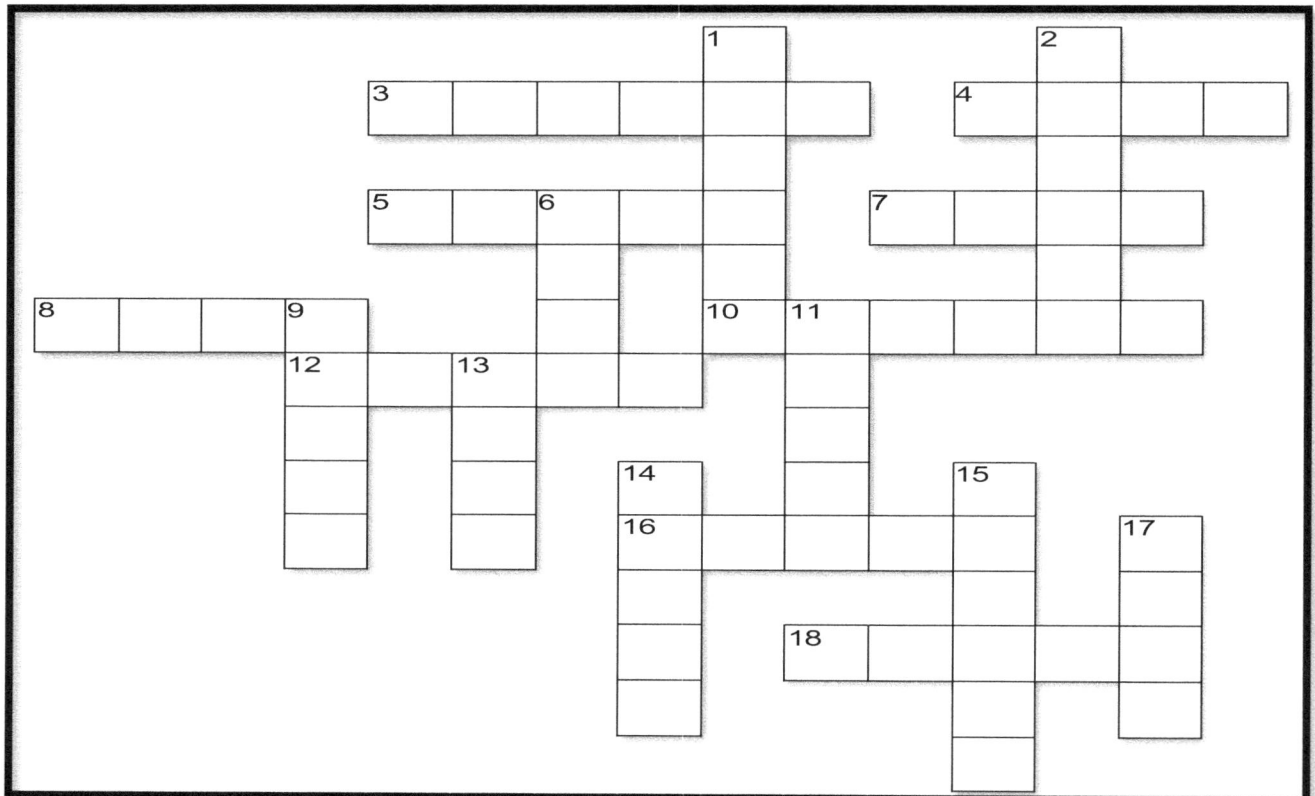

MEGA- PUZZLE CLUE

The first letter of # 13 answer is the letter for the Mega Puzzle # 31, 85, 220 &
Give up? Solutions are on Pages 74 & 79.   257.

SWITCHEROO. SWITCH OUT THEN IN, ONE LETTER FROM EACH LISTED NON- MEDICAL WORD TO FORM A MEDICAL TERM.
EXAMPLE: YOUTH M O U T H.

ACROSS

2. YOUTH M O U T H
4. RIM
5. LUNGE
7. INCUR
9. RIVER
10. KNEW

DOWN

1. MINUS
3. TALUK
6. SKIP
8. SERVE

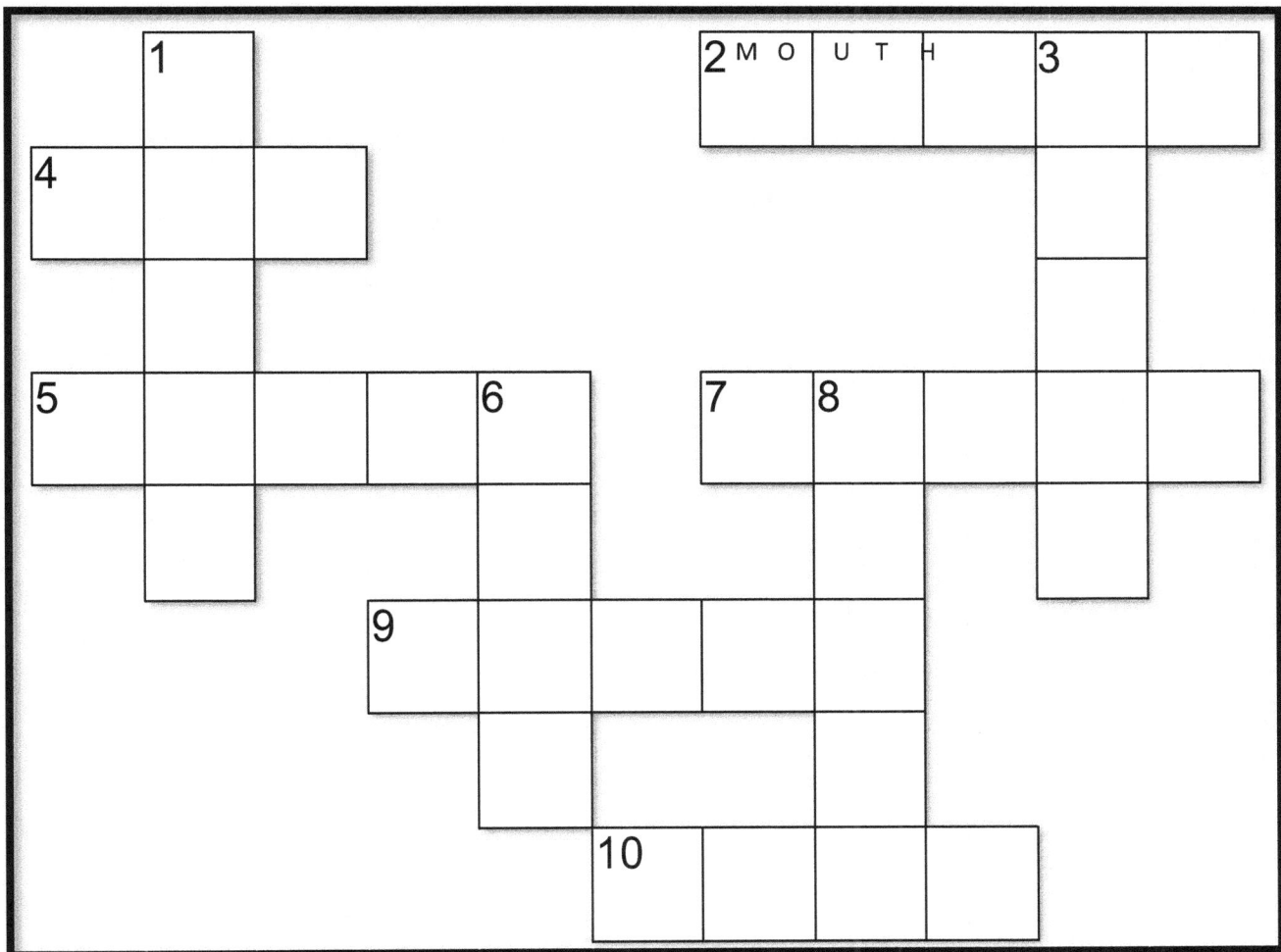

MEGA- PUZZLE CLUE

The first letter of # 1 answer is the letter for the Mega Puzzle # 288, 304, 310, 314, 320 & 326.

Give up? Solutions are on Pages 74 & 80.

INSERT THE MISSING LETTER FOR EACH LISTED WORD AND THEN LOCATE ALL THE WORDS ON THE GRID.

SOUND ALIKE WORDS

AFFERENT - EFFERENT

APHAGIA -   APHA _ IA

COLOSTRUM -   C _ AUSTRUM

CORD -   C _ ORD

DEPENDENT - DEPEND _ NT

DYSPHAGIA -   DYSPHA _ IA

ENURESIS -   _ NURESIS

ELICIT -   _ LLICIT

HUMERAL -   HUM _ RAL

ILEUM -   IL _ UM

PERFUSION -   P _ OFUSION

PERINEAL - PER _ NEAL

PLURAL - PL _ URAL

PROSTATE -   PROST _ ATE

```
N A L F Y D         B F R I D U
E M H I A A Y C     M I M L U M D D
M A C R L G R M A H   S I S E R U N E Y I
T N E R E F F A O E N O I S U F O R P P S B N
H B I G Z O I Z H M U P R M L A F E R E P X E
I I L K Y B R L L P U R E D X Y N T O N H U Z
S I S E R U N A I G A H P S Y D I A S D A Z K
P L K B I J Y E M U R T S U A L C T T E S I B
 E D Q W B H P P X M M Q N L A X S R N I L
 R F N E F F E R E N T I U R X O A T A
 O M U R T S O L O C X Z U P R T R
 N P E R F U S I O N D L U P E
 E L I C I T P R Y E P S M
 A W N I Y P D U A X U
 L A E N I R E P H
 A I S A H P A
 S L E I Z
 U R E
```

BONUS

O _ _ _ _ _ _

The last seven unused letters
reveal a word.

Give up? Solutions are on Pages 74 & 80.

MEGA- PUZZLE CLUE
The letter that is circled in
the bonus word is the Mega
Puzzle letter for # 122,125,126 & 137.

51

Chapter 13

Bones

FOLLOW THE ARROWS TO FIND THE BONES OF THE HEAD. EACH BONE HAS FOUR CLUES; THE NO OF LETTERS, THE FIRST AND LAST LETTER, AND A SPECIFICATION OR LOCATION OF THE BONE.

						8 P L		5 I S			8 S D	
6 C A	6 S S				Stirrup Shaped						Anvil Shaped
			9 Z C								
		5 H D				Horse- shoe Shaped				
8 T L						AKA Temple				
8 L L										
7 M A			Upper Jaw Bone			9 O L			Houses the Cribiform Plate	
Inferior Nasal...		7 E D					Bat/Butt er- fly Shaped	6 M S	
8 P E	Skull Roof		5 V R						
		Relates to the Palate	Cheek- bone					
5 N L		Nose Bridge	8 M E				Lower Jaw Bone	
Smallest Facial Bone	7 F L				Fore- head		
	Plough Shaped		Base of the Skull	Hammer shaped		

MEGA PUZZLE CLUE
The first letter of all the bones of the head that is most frequently occurring is the letter for the Mega Puzzle # 180, 295, 308, 322 & 324.

Give up? Solution is on Page 74.

FOLLOW THE ARROWS TO FIND THE BONES OF THE UPPER LIMB.

MEGA PUZZLE CLUE

The vowel that is least frequently occurring (on the grid) is the letter

for the Mega Puzzle # 179, 187, 192, 201, 204, 208, 210, 216, 223, 229,

234 & 240.

Give up? Solution is on Page 74.

FOLLOW THE ARROWS TO FIND THE BONES OF THE LOWER LIMB.

MEGA PUZZLE CLUE

The vowel that is least frequently occurring (on the grid) is the letter for the Mega Puzzle # 253, 256, 262, 269, 272, 275, 303, 307, 313, 328 & 330.

Give up? Solution is on Page 75.

Chapter 14

Joints

FOLLOW THE ARROWS TO FIND THE JOINTS OF THE UPPER LIMB.

12
G
L

Elbow
&
Wirst
Joint

17
A
R

11
H
R

16
S
R

10
R
R

16
C
L

15
I
L

15
I
L

11
I
L

11
R
L

19
M
L

AKA
MCP Joint
Of The
Hands

AKA
Shoulder
Joint

AKA
Trochlear
Joint
- Elbows

-Plane
Joint
Of The
Hands

AKA
Wrist Joint

AKA
CMC Joint
Of the
Hands

-Two Sets
DIP/PIP
Of The
Hand

AKA- AC
Joint
Of The
Shoulder

Plane
Joint
Of The
Hands

AKA SC
Joint
Of The
Shoulder

MEGA PUZZLE CLUE

The last letter of the shortest word (on the grid) is the letter for the Mega Puzzle # 273, 276, 300 & 312.

Give up? Solution is on Page 75.

FOLLOW THE ARROWS TO FIND THE JOINTS.

MEGA- PUZZLE CLUE

The first letter of the longest word (on the grid) is the letter for the Mega Puzzle # 284, 298 & 305.

Give up? Solution is on Page 75.

Chapter 15

The Three Ps Of Medicine

FIND THE PATHOLOGIES. THE NUMBERED LETTERS IN THE TABLE BELOW AND THE GRID ARE THE SAME. ENTER THE LETTERS IN THE GRID UNTIL THE WORDS ARE REVEALED.

1 H	3 M	5 S	6 ?	7 R	8 L	9 F	10 K	11 C	12 ?	13 V
14 ?	15 D	16 T	17 ?	18 N	20 Y	21 B	22 G	23 P	25 ?	26 X

MEGA- PUZZLE CLUE

The grid letter # 6 is the letter for the Mega Puzzle # 3, 57, 64, 95, 124, 141, 147, 173, 184 &214.

Give up? Solution is on Page 75.

FIND THE PHYSIOLOGICAL TERMS. THE NUMBERED LETTERS IN THE TABLE BELOW AND THE GRID ARE THE SAME. ENTER THE LETTERS IN THE GRID UNTIL THE WORDS ARE REVEALED.

1	3	4	5	6	7	8	9	11	14	15
?	?	?	B	V	T	M	S	P	?	?

16	17	18	19	20	21	22	23	24	25	26
?	?	?	Y	O	G	L	E	X	?	?

Give up? Solution is on Page 75.

MEGA- PUZZLE CLUE
The grid letter # 4 is the letter for the Mega Puzzle
15, 23, 26, 28, 41, 44, 46, 60, 68, 74 & 81.

FIND THE MOST COMMONLY PRESCRIBED DRUGS. THE NUMBERED LETTERS IN THE TABLE BELOW AND THE GRID ARE THE SAME. ENTER THE LETTERS IN THE GRID UNTIL THE WORDS ARE REVEALED.

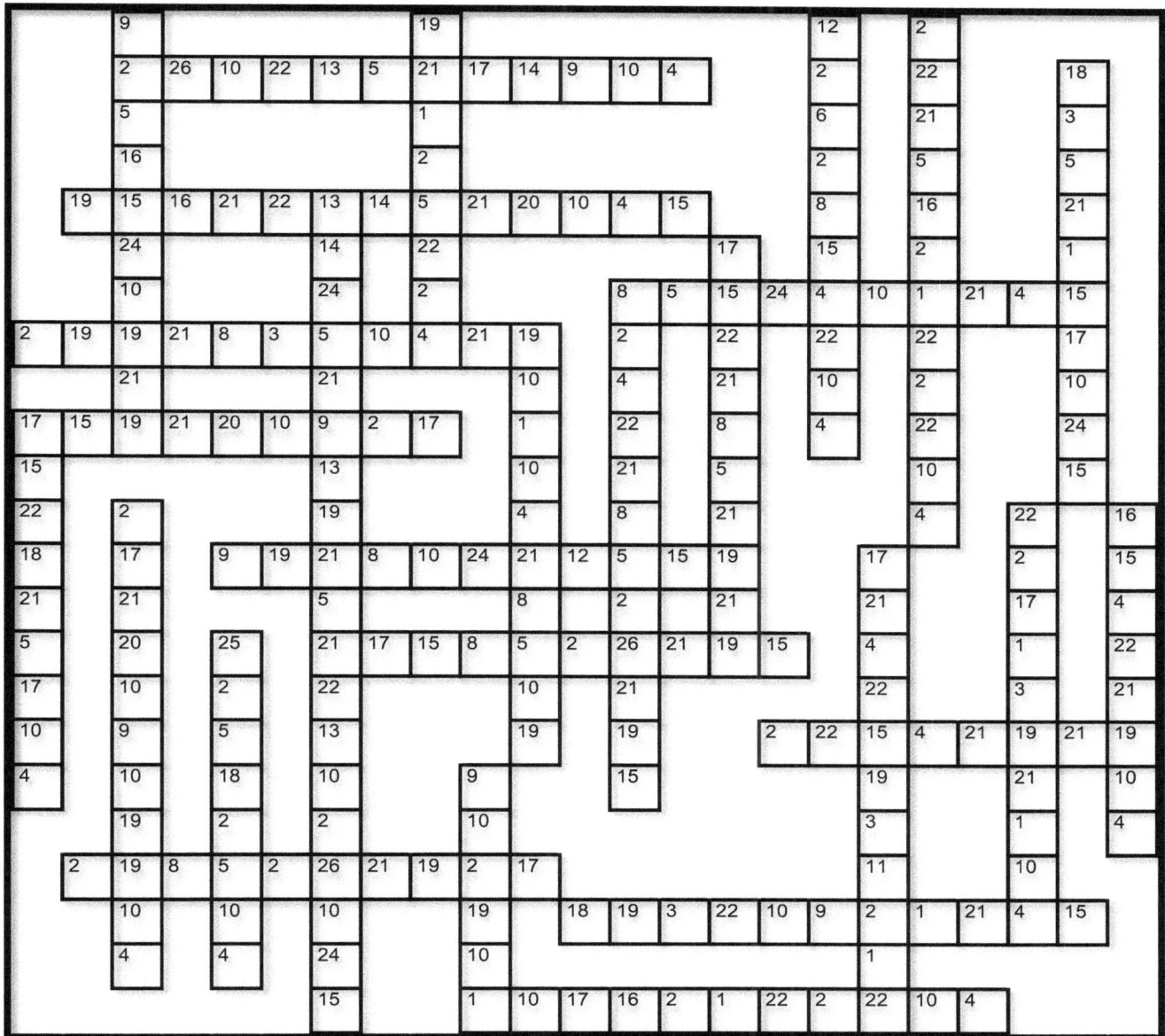

1 ?	2 A	3 U	4 N	5 R	6 B	8 P	9 ?	10 ?	11 ?	12 ?	13 ?
14 ?	15 E	16 V	17 M	18 F	19 L	20 X	21 ?	22 ?	24 ?	25 ?	26 ?

MEGA PUZZLE CLUE

The grid letter # 2 is the letter for the Mega Puzzle # 13, 35, 70, 86, 91, 107, 131, 151, 157, 164 & 176.

Give up? Solution is on Pages 75 & 80.

Chapter 16

Misspelled Words

INCORRECTLY SPELLED WORDS AND ABBREVIATIONS

ELEPHANTITIS E L E P H A N T I A S I S
FIBERMANALGIA _ _ _ _ _ _ _ _ _ _ _ _ _
GABBAGANTIN _ _ _ _ _ _ _ _ _ _
GULLBLADDER _ _ _ _ _ _ _ _ _ _
GLUCASAUSAGE _ _ _ _ _ _ _ _ _ _
ANESCEASIA _ _ _ _ _ _ _ _ _ _
ALBUTIROL _ _ _ _ _ _ _ _ _
AMIROADERONE _ _ _ _ _ _ _ _ _ _
HEINEKIN _ _ _ _ _ _ _ _
HYMNOPTOSIS _ _ _ _ _ _ _ _ _ _

FORCEMIDE _ _ _ _ _ _ _ _ _ _
ATENENOL _ _ _ _ _ _ _ _
AUGIEMENTIM _ _ _ _ _ _ _ _ _
CABBAGE _ _ _ _
CANADA _ _ _ _ _ _ _
CAPNEOGRAPHY _ _ _ _ _ _ _ _ _ _ _
CATILLAC _ _ _ _ _ _ _ _
CELLULITITIS _ _ _ _ _ _ _ _ _ _
CHLOROLESTERAL _ _ _ _ _ _ _ _ _ _ _
HEROINE _ _ _ _ _ _

DIAREAH _ _ _ _ _ _ _ _
DEFIBULATOR _ _ _ _ _ _ _ _ _ _ _ _ _
HTCZ _ _ _ _
HYENA _ _ _ _ _ _
HYDRAZALINE _ _ _ _ _ _ _ _ _ _
AMBALANCE _ _ _ _ _ _ _ _ _
AMARYSM _ _ _ _ _ _ _ _
ARTHURITIS _ _ _ _ _ _ _ _ _
DIABETIS _ _ _ _ _ _ _ _

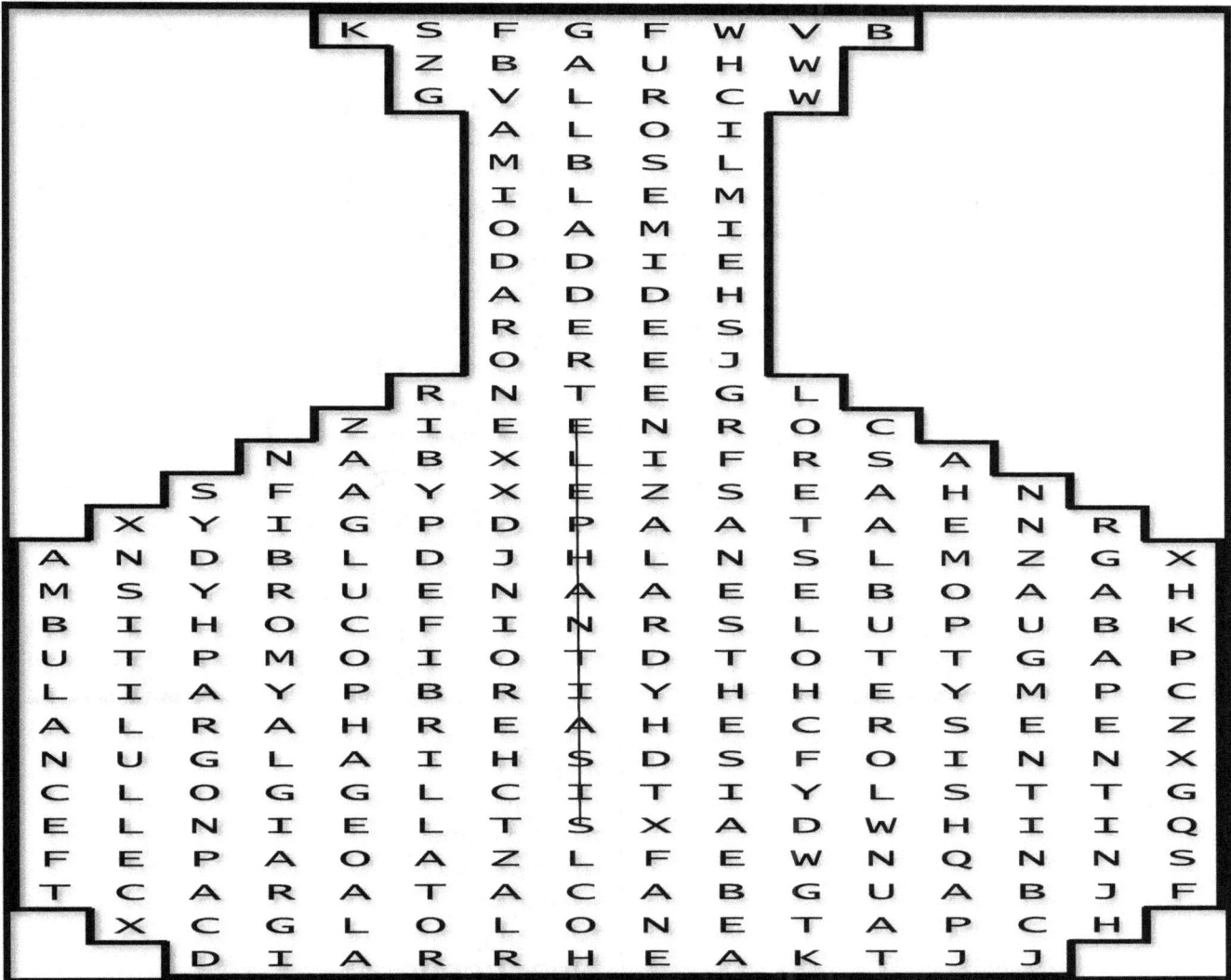

```
              K S F G F W V   B
                Z B A U H W   W
                G V L R C W   W
                A L O I
                M B S L
                I L E M
                O A M I
                D D I E
                A D D H
                R E D S
                O R E J
              R N T E G   L
            Z I E E N R   O C
          N A B X I F R   S A
        S F A Y X S E A   H N       R
      X Y I G P D P A T A E N       R
    A N D B L D J H L N S L M Z G   X
    M S Y R U E N A E E B O A A H
    B I H O C F I N R S L U P U B K
    U T P M O I O T D T O T T G A P
    L I A Y P B R I Y H H E Y M P C
    A L R A H R E A H E C R S E E Z
    N U G L A I H S D S F O I N X
    C L O G G L C I T I Y L S T T G
    E L I E L T S X A D W H I I Q
    F E P A O A Z L F E W N Q N N S
    T C A R A T A C A B G U A B J F
      X C G L O L O N E T A P C H
        D I A R R R H E A K T J J
```

FIND THE CORRECT SPELLING FOR EACH LISTED INCORRECTLY SPELLED WORD AND ABBREVIATION.

Give up? Solutions are on Pages 76 & 80.

FIND THE CORRECT SPELLING FOR EACH LISTED INCORRECTLY SPELLED WORD AND ABBREVIATION.

Bonus

Ο̶ _ _ _ _ _

The last six unused letters in his left foot
reveal a word.

```
O L Y           W P E Z
P R Y H         P H L A N N
E R N Y O       P R C I N N
  O N O   P       R Y L S
  Z O   P   D R I Q   F O V S   X Q Z   H
  K     K R O A A   O P G S I   U A G R A   Y
                C A N O P O T   Y F S   N A H D F I   H I Q D Y
                K O O R P R L   L S S   T U
                P P R P D K   Y M L H
                V R P S C X O   M
              P I P N H O D B   I B N
              P L O C J L   B A B U I D
                O S E C A D T S   H R C   P N
                A C H I L L E S Z U   N W   R O I D
                L A N I M O D B       B   F A M
                Z J B Z   R Q A U       W   E N U O C   G O
                                        W   P E N       N
```

INCORRECTLY SPELLED WORDS

IBUBUFFERIN _ _ _ _ _ _ _ _ _   VICKODE _ _ _ _ _ _ _

LASIK _ _ _ _ _   VESICAL _ _ _ _ _ _

ABOMINABLE _ _ _ _ _ _ _ _ _   PROPOTHOL _ _ _ _ _ _ _ _

AKILESE _ _ _ _ _ _ _   PROPANOLOL _ _ _ _ _ _ _ _ _ _ _

COODAMIN _ _ _ _ _ _ _ _   PROLOSEX _ _ _ _ _ _ _ _

VIAGRY _ _ _ _ _   RHABDOMYOLITIS _ _ _ _ _ _ _ _ _ _ _ _ _

HYDROCORDONE _ _ _ _ _ _ _ _ _ _ _ _

MEGA- PUZZLE CLUE

The LETTER THAT IS CIRCLED IN THE BONUS WORD

is the Mega Puzzle letter for # 6, 8, 18, 21, 115, 120 & 136.

Give up? Solutions are on Pages 76 & 80.

INCORRECTLY SPELLED WORDS

DIAGNOSISES _ _ _ _ _ _ _ _ _ _

HEFARIN _ _ _ _ _ _ _

DRYALYSIS _ _ _ _ _ _ _ _ _

DIALASIZE _ _ _ _ _ _ _

RISPERIDAL _ _ _ _ _ _ _ _ _ _

AMTRACKS _ _ _ _ _ _ _

REFLEX _ _ _ _ _ _ _

NAUSEAOUAS _ _ _ _ _ _ _ _ _

SKEZURES _ _ _ _ _ _ _ _

WINGWORMS _ _ _ _ _ _ _ _ _ _

PREGNISONE _ _ _ _ _ _ _ _ _ _

ANTIBEOTICS _ _ _ _ _ _ _ _ _ _ _ _

TENDERNITIS _ _ _ _ _ _ _ _ _ _

THRASH _ _ _ _ _ _ _

UMBIBLICAL _ _ _ _ _ _ _ _ _ _

VIRGINAL _ _ _ _ _ _ _ _

VERTAGO _ _ _ _ _ _ _

HICKERECTOMY _ _ _ _ _ _ _ _ _ _ _ _

SCHITZOPHRENIA _ _ _ _ _ _ _ _ _ _ _ _ _ _

CHOIRPRACTER _ _ _ _ _ _ _ _ _ _ _ _

BUPROPRION _ _ _ _ _ _ _ _ _

FIND THE CORRECT SPELLING FOR EACH LISTED INCORRECTLY SPELLED WORD AND ABBREVIATION.

```
            A N T H R A X
            I O E Y O N U
            N I N S T T L
            E P D T C I F
            R O O E A B E
            H R N R R I R
U F W X F S P P I E P O G I T R E V R
B W E O R X O U T C O T H R U S H O A
K C N F X D Z B I T R I N G W O R M S
B S E R U Z I E S O I C D D C M P C B
V O H P C M H A P M H S I N V R W D X
U M B I L I C A L Y C A A A E Y J B E
L A D R E P S I R Y L U G D E O A E O
            H T E Y S I N
            W K Z E N I O
            O E O A S F S
            X U L O M O E
            S D N N I Y S
            H E P A R I N
```

Give up? Solutions are on Pages 76 & 80.

INCORRECTLY SPELLED WORDS

MENAPAUSE _ _ _ _ _ _ _ _ _

PERSCRIBE _ _ _ _ _ _ _ _ _

ANTICUBICAL _ _ _ _ _ _ _ _ _ _ _

MEXOTREXATE _ _ _ _ _ _ _ _ _ _ _ _

ANTIBEOTIC _ _ _ _ _ _ _ _ _ _

EDEMINOUS _ _ _ _ _ _ _ _ _

METOPROPOL _ _ _ _ _ _ _ _ _ _

OSTEOSPEROSIS _ _ _ _ _ _ _ _ _ _ _ _

CIPROFLUCLOXACILLEN _ _ _ _ _ _ _ _ _ _ _ _ _ _ _

OPTHALMOLOGY _ _ _ _ _ _ _ _ _ _ _ _

PERSCRIPTION _ _ _ _ _ _ _ _ _ _ _ _

FIND THE CORRECT SPELLING FOR EACH LISTED INCORRECTLY SPELLED WORD AND ABBREVIATION.

```
                    W G I
                  B U R R S E M
                E S U O T A M E D E I
              G Y P I L E X T N I O W I
            D Y Y K V F I O I X N R M P W
            J A X L R V P T X S I R A R M
          P P R E S C R I B E P C K N E E K
          L R C I T O I B I T N A M T S N Z
        V W M S F L Q B S L P L X H E C O Q P
        Y G O L O M L A H T H P O X C R P E X
        V F J L M R H Q Y S X T L Z U I A F I
          H O G E Q T Y E E R P F P B P U O
          S I S O R O P O E T S O M I T S K
            X F N D Z Q X D A R R C T I E
            Z O O L T A P O B C P U A O Y
              T K J T F W C U J I I L N
                P E C X F P V Q C A D
    BONUS           S T E R N U T
    _ _ _ _ _ _ _ _ _ _     A T E
The last ten unused letters reveal a word.
```

MEGA- PUZZLE CLUE
The letter that is circled in the bonus word
Is the mega puzzle letter for # 236, 249, 260, 292, 294 & 323.

Give up? Solutions are on Pages 76 & 80.

General Medicine Word Games

1a

N	X	V	E	R	T	E	B	R	A	E	D
E	A	V	I	T	C	N	U	J	N	O	C
E	V	C	T	E	J	Y	W	E	L	Q	M
A	L	E	B	G	A	G	A	K	G	P	M
S	T	A	N	W	F	L	X	K	E	P	J
R	P	R	K	A	U	Q	L	T	H	T	F
U	C	E	L	P	E	T	E	I	W	L	G
B	R	L	A	G	J	C	H	N	X	Z	B
D	R	C	R	M	H	P	A	N	R	A	N
R	S	S	V	I	K	T	M	V	N	M	G
L	H	L	A	M	T	C	D	N	A	R	H
K	T	E	E	R	M	N	P	K	Y	E	R

2b

N	S	I	S	A	T	S	A	T	E	M	K
Z	M	N	M	A	N	A	L	Y	S	I	S
W	D	D	S	F	Y	L	J	I	F	W	S
E	P	I	K	I	W	P	S	X	R	X	I
X	R	B	A	L	T	O	T	E	M	S	S
O	O	J	M	G	R	S	P	K	S	I	I
S	N	Y	K	U	N	A	E	I	T	V	R
T	N	H	E	C	T	O	R	T	J	L	H
O	O	N	L	I	G	I	S	W	P	E	T
S	S	V	T	W	N	T	Q	I	J	P	R
I	I	I	T	B	Y	T	T	M	S	Y	X
S	S	S	I	M	Y	D	I	D	I	P	E

4a

C	K	M	T	A	C	L	Y	A	R	A
O	H	T	G	T	Q	D	T	S	C	T
N	Y	R	V	A	T	A	N	A	R	A
D	F	X	Z	M	M	R	K	R	M	M
Y	K	M	J	O	T	J	M	C	A	O
L	Q	K	N	Y	J	R	X	O	M	N
O	V	E	K	M	K	T	K	M	O	I
M	D	S	T	O	M	A	T	A	R	C
A	J	J	D	I	P	G	R	T	B	R
T	L	R	L	E	B	N	L	A	I	A
A	B	N	L	U	H	D	K	J	F	C

1b

A	R	F	S	C	L	E	R	A	A	A
C	V	K	P	R	D	R	H	R	Y	L
H	N	I	W	E	F	X	B	T	Q	L
A	V	K	T	W	T	E	Z	J	L	I
V	L	R	P	C	T	E	S	J	L	A
A	R	L	T	R	N	C	C	L	R	
C	R	L	E	P	A	U	Y	H	Q	N
A	V	V	T	P	K	X	J	B	I	T
N	A	G	U	H	K	W	Y	N	D	A
E	D	L	A	S	R	U	B	K	O	N
V	A	W	X	R	K	C	V	W	C	C

3a

Q	M	C	P	L	G	W	W	B	J
K	Y	T	E	L	M	S	K	R	S
R	C	N	R	R	J	E	K	E	L
Q	L	T	N	P	V	C	C	L	F
V	A	R	I	C	E	I	X	C	Z
D	L	Q	H	Y	T	D	C	Z	N
W	D	V	Q	R	M	N	M	E	F
M	Y	G	O	T	N	I	V	Y	S
S	E	C	I	D	N	E	P	P	A
B	F	O	R	N	I	C	E	S	X

4b

Z	P	C	J	R	N	Q	A	A	A
M	N	A	C	A	Q	S	M	M	M
N	J	R	F	M	W	A	O	O	O
W	S	C	I	B	O	L	L	Y	Y
J	T	I	B	N	D	C	Y	D	M
J	N	N	R	E	M	O	D	N	O
N	M	O	O	D	D	M	N	O	I
Q	A	M	M	F	A	A	A	O	E
H	K	A	A	W	Y	R	C	L	L

2a

K	E	P	I	D	I	D	Y	M	I	D	E	S	H
K	R	X	R	E	X	O	S	T	O	S	E	S	D
G	Y	P	B	S	L	H	P	J	E	K	X	E	I
F	H	R	R	T	E	D	J	D	B	N	N	S	A
X	E	L	P	O	K	V	I	Q	E	L	Q	O	G
F	P	T	G	Z	G	X	R	L	U	V	S	J	N
L	A	N	K	R	I	N	R	E	E	N	H	R	O
Y	R	I	S	L	R	Z	O	O	S	P	T	R	S
R	I	E	T	B	Q	S	W	S	K	T	P	E	E
X	T	T	E	R	L	W	V	E	K	T	S	R	
X	D	S	T	A	G	N	P	K	S	Z	P	C	
C	E	T	A	H	H	Z	M	R	G	R	Q	W	Z
Y		S	E	S	A	T	S	A	T	E	M	N	H

3b

C	H	L	P	X	T	A	C
T	T	S	I	X	A	P	E
A	U	R	F	I	P	E	R
R	A	X	O	T	E	N	V
V	R	E	R	R	C	D	I
P	M	D	N	O	A	I	X
S	I	N	I	C	A	A
A	V	I	X	K	R	X	B

5a

L	K	X	Y	X	R	S	B	Y	S
S	S	L	X	S	B	A	N	A	G
A	A	L	T	H	T	M	M	R	J
M	M	F	I	B	R	O	M	A	S
O	N	C	B	N	L	M	D	N
C	E	B	M	I	Q	Y	N	A	N
R	L	C	Q	F	D	D	F	S
A	D	R	Y	J	G	N	L	L
S	A	M	O	Y	M	O	I	E	L
C	B	L	N	W	M	C	V	P	Y

69

5b

7a

8b

6a

7b

9a

6b

8a

9b

10a

11b

14

10b

12

15

11a

13

16

17

20

23

18

21

24

19

4	9	8	5	6	2	1	3	7
1	7	6	8	3	9	4	5	2
2	3	5	1	7	4	6	8	9
3	5	2	9	8	6	7	4	1
7	8	1	2	4	5	9	6	3
9	6	4	7	1	3	5	2	8
6	4	7	3	9	8	2	1	5
5	1	3	4	2	7	8	9	6
8	2	9	6	5	1	3	7	4

22

25

26

```
Q W C T U G R Q Z R M A R D
W Z V M A A Q W X L I Q S A
E X B E S S S E C K A G D S
R C N T D D Q R B S S E S D
T V N S F F D A L Q T W S F
Y B H Q Q G F C R W D R S G
U N N W D G A B A S F R S H
I M D F F P A O S G T F D
I N A A L G G T P E B Y G F
O B I S G H Y O R F I J G
P V S I C D Q U I A G T S H
L C Q D D C R I S H R J H
J F W R U O R I D A T H J
N S T E M I M P U S J Y G O
```

29

```
T W E R I L U I O M B P L K S
F E G L B N Y D U F G I H T J
F G E G Z X C M V B N M O K L
K U J T H A P G P B F M G Q L
M A S S H S T S U H A D F G D
C Z X C S V B X M N R J P L S
A R S H D F S G H J E I K
Q W O V E A R L T A R A X L U
T C Y U A U A I O P L U N I K
K J H G P R F D S A S Z A X S
C C P V T B I N M M G L H K C
P Q Q A O I U X A Y T H R E E
H U Y Q G H J K I K L F L S J
S J S K N J K J C K T J K J
```

32

TESTS OVARY SKI ATRI
STOMACH KIDNEY PANCREAS
PITUITARY THYROID PARATHYROID
DUODENUM

27

```
N D G Q W F M H E S I D S F F
S F G T E G C R R S T R A V G
F F N U H O H S D R I R F F
E R F B E G K H T A C L S F
M G T T R H R C Y F R T C G G
I R S S T O G Q R G Y G I F G
A G T Y S H F W Y O H H D G F
P O C A J S E U J T H N H G
C G H Y D R D R U H C J A H D
U H Y U A J A T I Q T N P F D
I J J S F J H Y K W P N D I C
S R K S G K H E J E R N F D D
D J D S H L G Y L R G A H D F
F H P S J L H U A L H D L F H
G G F H K O J I S T P C O S G
```

30

PNEUMOPERITONEUM DERMATOMYOSITIS
GRAVES HYPOGLYCEMIA MELANOMA
PREGNANCY HYPOCALCEMIA SARCOIDOSIS
DIPHTHERIA HERPES CHOLECYSTITIS PERITONITIS MEASLES APPENDICITIS
MENINGITIS MUMPS
SACROILIITIS PERICARDITIS
GOUT TRYPANOSOMIASIS
SPLENOMEGALY

33

NERVOUS LYMPHATIC RESPIRATORY
MUSCULAR SKELETAL PROOROUT
DIGESTIVE URINARY
CARDIOVASCULAR
ENDOCRINE
INTEGUMENTARY

28

```
Y A T F A N E Y U L E R E W D
G P H G I P U R P M R P M E S
O L O H N O M A N O U T A R D
M W E J G E R T Y L S S E M Q
L Q W E F D D B N D D E M B W
O G S D D F U A O A U N A R E
I F D D R D C T L T C A A R R
U D S D E S R T R O T L V I T
E A L A R I A H E S O L E C Y
S E D R T T I R N I N D S A
D O H R H I N H S S E M I D G
F N N H H S E P D H O S O N
Q O I I F N N F E S Y L S E P
W T I B F O I E F F G S I H A
W E R T G I T C G G F D T I T
```

31

METHEMOGLOBINEMIA
PARACETAMOL INSULIN ORGANOPHOSPHATE
SULFONYLUREA THALLIUM IRON
BENZODIAZEPINE WARFARIN LEAD
METHOTREXATE
ISONIAZID DIGOXIN
CYANIDE

34

BREAST KNEE SKIN NERVE
HEART LUNG TEETH
MOUTH JOINT RIB ATRIA PENIS
TENDON SINUS

35

```
          T           R
LUMBAR   HEAD
          R           T
PENIS     I    SKIN   N
          O           A
BONE      D    SACRAL
   LIVER       T
   B           R    U
   O   I   T   I    T
   W   N   H   HEART  K
          I    U      N
          G    NERVE  E
          H    U      E
               S
```

36

```
S              MOUTH
R I B          A
I              L
N   LUNGS      INCUS
S       K      E    U
   LIVER   N   V    S
        N      V
         KNEE
```

37

38

```
    STAPES   INCUS
 C       A   Z        P
 O       R   HYOID    H
 N       I   Y        E
 C       TEMPORAL     N
 H       T   M        O
 MAXILLA L   ETHMOID  I
    A    A   I   C    M
    C    L   C   C    A
 PALATINE  V     I    L
    R    I  O    P    L
    I    N  E    I    E
 NASAL  E   MANDIBLE  U
    L       E   T     S
            FRONTAL
            L
```

39

```
         TRAPEZIUM
              H
   TRIQUETRAL      S
 T                 C    M
 R HAMATE    CAPITATE   E
 A       P   N     P    T
 P       C   G     H    A
 E       L   E     O    C
 Z  RADIUS   U     I    A
 O       V   L     D    R
 I       I   N          P
 D       C   RM  SCAPULA  A
         L              L
 LUNATE      HUMERUS
```

40

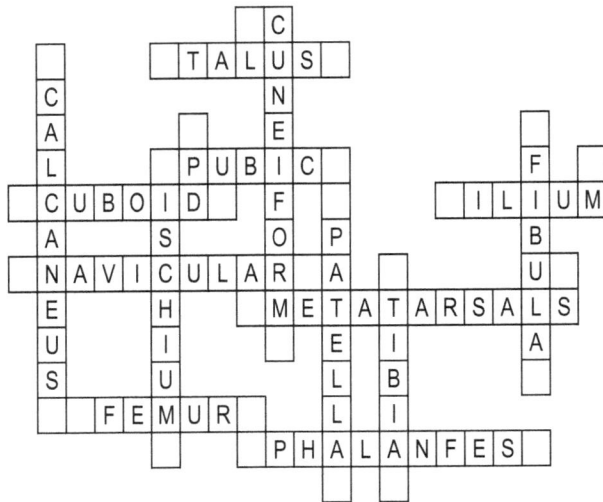

41

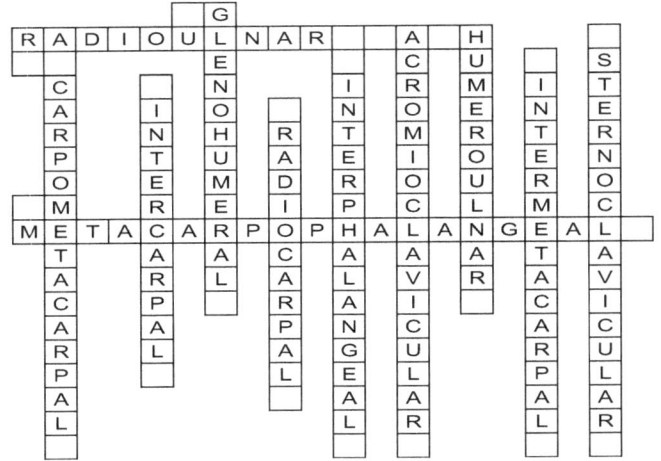

42

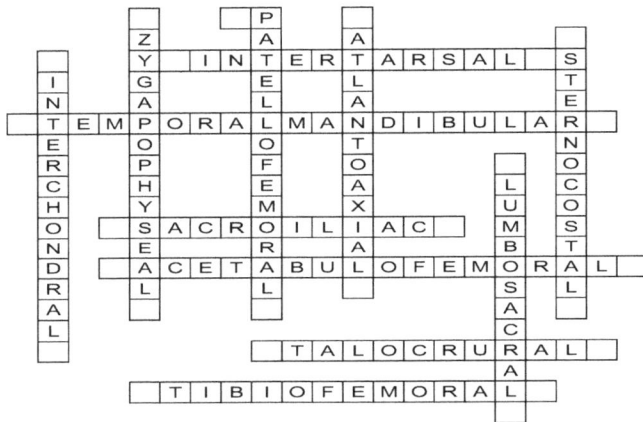

43

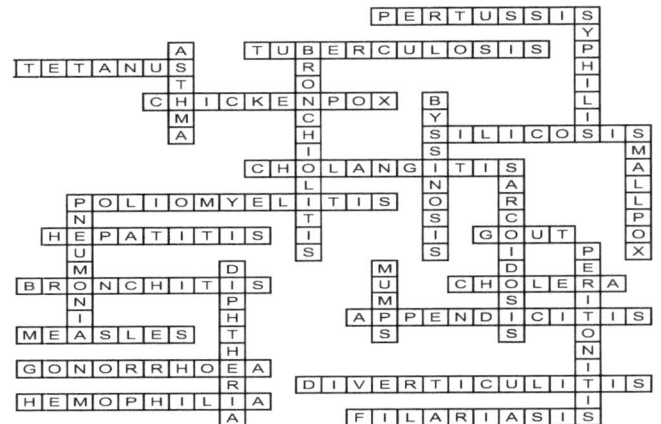

44

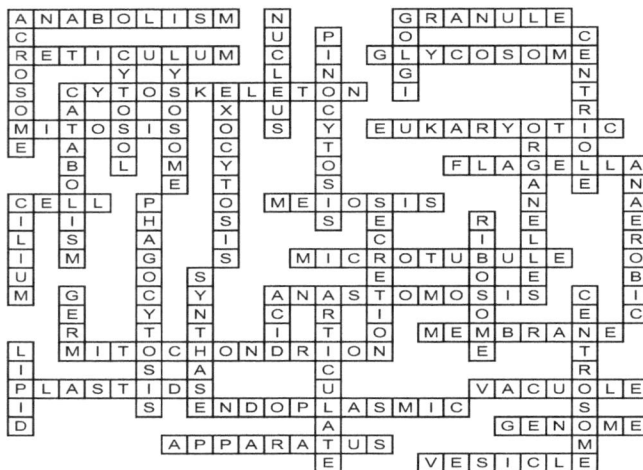

45

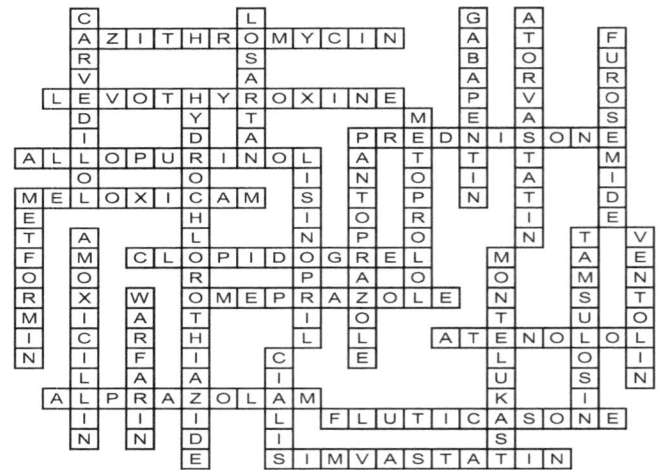

46

47

48

49

Puzzles # 1a & 1b

axilla axillae
bursa bursae/ bursas
conjunctiva conjunctivae
larva larvae
petechia petechiae
scapula scapulae / scapulas
sclera sclerae / scleras
vena cava venae cavae
vertebra vertebrae

Puzzles # 2a & 2b

analysis analyses
arthrosis arthroses
diagnosis diagnoses
exostosis exostoses
metastasis metastases
neurosis neuroses
pelvis pelves/ pelvises
prognosis prognoses
testis testes
Exceptions:
epididymis epididymides
Iris irides / irises
hepatitis hepatitides /
hepatitises

Puzzles # 3a & 3b

appendix appendices /
appendixes
cervix cervices

cortex cortices
fornix fornices
index indices / indexes
varix varices

Puzzles # 4a & 4b

adenoma adenomata
carcinoma carcinomata
condyloma condylomata
fibroma fibromata
leiomyoma leiomyomata
sarcoma sarcomata
stoma stomata

Puzzles # 5a & 5b

adenoma adenomas
carcinoma carcinomas
condyloma condylomas
fibroma fibromas
leiomyoma leiomyomas
sarcoma sarcomas
stoma stomas

Puzzles # 6a & 6b

larynx larynges
meninx meninges
phalanx phalanges

Puzzles # 7a & 7b

acetabulum acetabula /
acetabulums
antrum antra
atrium atria
bacterium bacteria
diverticulum diverticula
endocardium endocardia
ileum ilea
labium labia
medium media
myocardium myocardia /
myocardiums
ovum ova
septum septa

Puzzles # 8a & 8b

bronchus bronchi
calculus calculi
coccus cocci
digitus digiti
embolus emboli
esophagus esophagi
fungus fungi
glomerulus glomeruli
meniscus menisci
nucleus nuclei / nucleuses

Exceptions

corpus corpora
plexus plexuses
sinus sinuses
virus viruses

viscus viscera

Puzzles # 9a & 9b

bronchoscope-
bronchoscopes
disease diseases
endoscope endoscopes
finger fingers
gland glands
tendon tendons
vein veins

Puzzles # 10a & 10b

artery arteries
biopsy biopsies
bronchoscopy -
bronchoscopies
cardiomyopathy -
cardiomyopathies
deformity deformities
ovary ovaries
therapy therapies

Puzzles # 11a & 11b

abscess abscesses
bypass bypasses
crutch crutches
patch patches

Puzzles # 12, 14, & 16

abdomen abdominal
adnexa adnexal
alveolus alveolar
anatomy anatomical
antrum antral
anus anal
aorta aortic
appendix appendiceal
arm brachial
artery arterial
aryepiglotticus aryepiglottic
atrium atrial
bladder vesical
bone osseous
brachium brachial
bronchus bronchial
cecum cecal
cerebrum cerebral
cervix cervical
clitoris clitoral
coitus coital
commissure commissural
cranium cranial
cuticle cuticular
cutis cutaneous
cytology cytological
decidua decidual
dermis dermal
dorsum dorsal
duodenum duodenal
dura dural
ear aural
embryo embryonic
esophagus esophageal
ethmoid ethmoidal
eye ocular
face facial
fascia fascial
feces fecal
fibula fibular

focus focal
foetus foetal
foot pedal
gestation gestational
gingiva gingival
gland glandular
glottis glottic
gluteus gluteal
gonad gonadal
gyrus gyral
heart cardiac
hemiplegia hemiplegic
hernia hernial
hiatus hiatal
hypophysis hypophyseal
hypothalamus hypothalamic
ileum ileal
ilium iliac
intestine intestinal
ischium ischial
jejunum jejunal
labium labial
larynx laryngeal
lethargy lethargic
leukocyte leukocytic
mania manic
maxilla maxillary
medicine medical
meninges meningeal
metaphysis metaphyseal
mouth oral
mucus mucosal
omentum omental
orbit orbital
ovary ovarian
pelvis pelvic
penis penile
pia pial
prostate prostatic
rectum rectal
spine spinal

spleen splenic
thymus thymic
tongue lingual
trachea tracheal
ureter ureteral / ureteric
uterus uterine
vagina vaginal
vein veinous
vertebra vertebral
virus viral

Puzzles # 13, 15, & 17

ACOU-: of or relating to hearing
ADEN-: of or pertaining to a gland
ADIP(O)-: of or relating to fat or fatty tissue
ADREN-: of or relating to adrenal glands
AMNI-: pertaining to the membranous fetal sac
ANGI-: pertaining to blood vessels
ANGIO-: related to blood vessels
ARTHR-: related to a joint
CARDI-: of or pertaining to the heart
CERVIC-: of or pertaining to the neck, the cervix
CHOL(E)-: of or pertaining to bile
COLONO-: related to large intestine colon
COLP(O)-: of or pertaining to the vagina
COLPO-: related to the vagina
COST- of or pertaining to the ribs
CYSTO-: related to the bladder
DENT-: of or pertaining to teeth
FACI-: of or pertaining to the face
GASTR-: related to stomach
GENU-: of or pertaining to the knee
GINGIV-: of or pertaining to the gum
GYNECO-: pertaining to the female genital
GYNO-: pertaining to female genital
HEMA-: of or pertaining to blood
HEPAT-: related to the liver
HYSTER(O)-: related to the uterus
LAPAR-: related to the abdominal cavity
MASTO-: related to the breast
OOPHOR-: related to the ovary
ORCHID-: related to the testicle
RHINO-: related to the nose

Puzzles # 25, 26, & 27

ACLS: advanced cardiac life support.
AIDS: acquired immune deficiency syndrome
CABG: coronary artery bypass graph
COPD: chronic obstructive pulmonary disease
DCIS: ductal carcinoma in situ

DIC: disseminated intravascular coagulation
DMARD: disease-modifying antirheumatic drug
GABA: gamma-aminobutyric acid
GERD: gastroesophageal reflux disease
HAART: highly active antiretroviral therapy
HADS: hospital anxiety and depression scale
HELLP: hemolysis, elevated liver enzyme, low platelets.
HOCM: hypertrophic obstructive cardiomyopathy
IRDS: infant respiratory distress syndrome
IUCD: intrauterine contraceptive devices
IUGR: intrauterine growth restriction
MCTD: mixed connective tissue disease.
MRSA: methicillin resistant staphylococcus aureus.
NSTEMI: non-ST- elevation myocardial infraction
PALS: pediatric advanced life support
PCOS: polycystic ovarian syndrome
PPTCT: prevention of parent-to-child transmission (of HIV)
PROM: premature rupture of membranes.
ROSC: return of spontaneous circulation
SARS: severe acute respiratory syndrome
SCID: severe combined immunodeficiency
SIADH: syndrome of inappropriate antidiuretic hormone
SIDS: sudden infant death syndrome
SIRS: systemic inflammatory response syndrome
SOAP: subjective, objective, assessment, plan
SSRI: selective serotonin reuptake inhibitor
SSSS: staphylococcus scalded skin syndrome

STEMI: ST-elevation myocardial infraction
TORCH: toxoplasmosis, others (syphilis, varicella-zoster, parvovirus b19), rubella, cytomegalovirus (cmv) and herpes infections

Puzzle 34

atria: latria
brain: bran
breast: beast
hair: air
heart: hear
incus: incuse
joint: join
knee: kneel
liver: sliver
lung: lunge
mouth: mouthy
nerve: nerved
penis: pens
rib: crib
sinus: sins
skin: skink
spine: spin
teeth: tebeth
tendon: tenon
testis: tests

Puzzle # 35

atria: tiara.
bone: ebon
elbow: below
head: hade
heart: earth,
knee: keen
liver: viler
lumbar: labrum
nerve: never
node: done
penis: pines, snipe.
retina: retain
sacral: rascal.
sclera: clears
skin: inks
tarsus: sutras
thigh: hight
 uterus: suture

Puzzle # 36

incus: incur

knee: knew

liver: river

lung: lunge

mouth: youth

nerve: serve

rib: rim

sinus: minus

skin: skip

talus: taluk

Puzzle # 37

afferent-efferent

aphagia-aphasia

colostrum-claustrum

cord-chord

dependent-dependant

dysphagia-dysphasia

elicit-illicit

enuresis-anuresis

humeral-humoral

ileum-ilium

perfusion-profusion

perineal-peroneal

pleural-plural

prostate-prostrate

Puzzle #45

Allopurinol

Alprazolam

Amoxicillin

Atenolol

Atorvastatin

Azithromycin

Carvedilol

Cialis

Clopidogrel

Fluticasone

Furosemide

Gabapentin

Hydrochlorothiazide

Levothyroxine

Lisinopril

Losartan

Meloxicam

Metformin

Metoprolol

Montelukast

Omeprazole

Pantoprazole

Prednisone

Simvastatin

Tamsulosin

Ventolin

Warfarin

Puzzles # 46, 47, 48, & 49

Abdominal -abominable

Achilles -akilese

Albuterol -albuterol

Ambulance ambalance

Amiodarone- amiroaderone

Anesthesia -anesceasia

Aneurysm-amarysm

Antecubital- anticubica

Anthrax-amtracks

Antibiotics- antibeolics

Arthritis-arthuritis

Atenolol-atenenol

Augmentin-augiementim

Bupropion- buproprion

CABG- cabbage

Candida - canada

Capnography capneography

Cataract-cadillac

Cellulitis-cellulititis

Chiropractor-choirpracter

Cholesterol -chlorolesteral

Ciprofloxacin- ciproflucloxacillen

Coumadin-coodamin

Defibrillator-defibulator

Diabetes -diabetis

Diagnoses- diagnosises

Dialysis-dryalysis

Dialyze- dialasize

Diarrhea -diareah

Edematous-edeminous

Elephantiasis-elephantitis

Fibromyalgia-fibermanalgia

Furosemide-forcemide

Gabapentin- gabbagantin

Gabapentin-gabbagantin

Gallbladder-gullbladder

Glucophage- glucasausage

HCTZ -htcz

Heimlich- heinekin

hemoptysis-hymnoptosis

Heparin-hefarin

Hernia-hyena

Heroin - heroine

Hydralazine-hydrazaline

Hydrocodone- hydrocordone

hysterectomy-hickerectomy

Ibuprofen- ibubufferin

Lasix-lasik

Menopause- menapause

Methotrexate-mexotrexate

Metoprolol-metopropol

Nauseous-nauseaouas

Ophthalmology-opthalmology

Osteoporosis -osteosperosis

Prednisone pregnisone

Prescribe-prescribe

Prescription-perscription

Prilosec- prolosex

Propofol-propothol

Propranolol- propanolol

Reflux-acid reflux

Rhabdomyolysis -rhabdomyolitis

Ringworms-wingworms

Risperdal-risperidal

Schizophrenia-schitzophrenia

Seizures-skezures

Seroquel-sequel

Tendonitis-tendernitis

Thrush-thrash

Umbilical- umbiblical

Vaginal - virginal

Vertigo-vertago

Vesicle- vesical

Viagra-viagry

Vicodin -vickode

www.ingramcontent.com/pod-product-compliance
Lightning Source LLC
Chambersburg PA
CBHW061618210326
41520CB00041B/7488